The Enemy in the Inner Me

Theresa Hart

ISBN-13: 978-0615667775
ISBN-10: 0615667775

Published by
Theresa Hart Books
www.authortheresahart.com

Printed in the United States of America.

This book is available at special quantity discounts for bulk purchase for sales promotions, fund-raising and educational needs. For information please write authortheresahart@gmail.com.

Cover Design by *Sehon Glynn*, SGrpahixs of NY
Author Photo by *Nicole Pope*

DISCLAIMER: All information has been portrayed as accurately as possible by the author. This book is not meant to diagnose, treat or heal any sickness or disease. It is a testimonial of one women's victory over cancer. Please consult your doctor if you have any type of health issue.

DEDICATION

I dedicate this book to all the cancer survivors and to all those who have won and are winning the victory over the enemy in the inner me.

CONTENTS

The Journey Continues...

ACKNOWLEDGMENTS

I first thank God, who is the Author and Finisher of my faith. Without God, I can do nothing, but with Him I can do all things through Christ that gives me strength. God has given me experience, time and wisdom to write this book.

Thank you ***Kevin Hart, my husband***, my best friend, my companion, who never left my side. You give true meaning to the wedding vows that say, "Do you promise to love her, comfort her, honor and keep her in sickness and in health, remaining faithful to her as long as you both shall live?" Thank you for loving me through it all. Through the years you have found something in me every day to fall in love with as I did you. Your strength and love has lifted and encouraged me to continue. NOBODY knows, but you and God, what it took to walk this walk. Our love continues to grow and that's why I love you so much. True love and devotion never dies; it lives forever.

To my daughter Nicole, a diamond in the rough who has blossomed into a radiant, beautiful woman. Seeing myself in you with everything I have taught you, but developing into your own woman – how fine is that. Thank you for being obedient and caring about what your parents think. I was the same way. You have developed into an awesome entrepreneur, mentor, and role model for young women. In today's times it's so needed for young people. Keep being you and don't let anybody change you, but God.

Mommy, you give new meaning to living life. Through your suffering mentally, emotionally, and most of all physically, you have managed to raise six beautiful children. Mommy, you have taught me that when you have the determination, and with God's help, you can endure to the end. I have never met a woman as strong as you. Love you, Mommy.

Thank you to my two baby brothers, Prince and Dupree. What strength I've received from you both during this time. The bible says the last shall be first and the first shall be last. You both have risen to the top against the status quo. The love I felt from you both is priceless. Love does what love is; it gives and that's what you both did. Thank you for being there.

To my son, Kevin, you are truly a blessing from God. Bishop Figueroa prophesied to me when I was pregnant with you in 1995. Bishop stated I would have a male child and that you would bring us much joy. God never lies. You have been a wonderful child from day one. Thank you for loving God first, loving your parents, loving your sister, and loving to do the right thing and striving for perfection in everything you do. Thank you for my hugs every day and our special times together; they are precious. You are a gift from God.

Thank you, North Shore Long Island Jewish Hospital Oncology, Hematology, and the Radiation Department, for being a big part of my recovery. God bless each and every one of you for doing your job with love, care, and affection.

Dorothy, I thank God for putting you in my life. You have been a blessing from day one. Thank you for helping with the proofing of my book. You have always helped me with my southern and broken English. I love you.

Maggie Pollydore, you are the woman I call my mother on the job. From the first day I met you, you staged my office and everything that I ever needed no matter what it was; whether it was for me or my family, you were there. I love you.

Jamesetta "Prophetess", thank you for being my friend, praying for me, giving me words of encouragement and being by my side when you didn't have to be. That's what friends are for. You have been up close and personal in my life from the first day I met you in the stairway on the job. God is going to send someone in your life to be there for you.

Thank you, ***Bishop Matthew Johnson and St. Albans Deliverance*** for praying, caring, and comforting me and my family while we were going through a testing time. God bless you all.

Gretchen Mitchell, thank you for never letting go. When I thought that was it, you called me on my job and said, "When are you coming home?" I will never forget it. Thanks for being the best writer I know and I was always privileged to be the first to read what you wrote. Thanks for sharing. Favor is coming to you so that the whole world will know who you are. "The last shall be first and the first shall be last."

I have the best co-workers in the whole wide world. God blessed me with people not just to work with, but to have a relationship with and that means a lot. Thank you to The Zucker Hillside Hospital.

To Bishop Eric R. Figueroa and First Lady Doreen Figueroa, thank you for always loving me and seeing the best in me when others saw the worst in me. Thank you for my growth and development in God. You both loved the pain out of me. You taught me how to trust God against all odds. It was you, Bishop, who said, "God is pushing this book out of you." and "You have suffered much, but God said He is going to give you double for your trouble." Thank you, Bishop Figueroa for being the voice of God to a hurting people; thank you to my New Life Tabernacle Family for loving me through pain and disappointment; you never gave up on me. Love really does cover a multitude of sins.

To my mother-in-law, Gladys Hart, my guardian Angel! I always felt like I was the daughter you never had. Thank you for your prayers, your sacrifices, your support, and for encouraging me to not give up.

To Junior, the artist of the cover of my book, to God be the Glory! I gave you the title of the book on the phone and through God's inspiration you put on paper what was in my heart. This cover says it all. Thank you for sharing your gift; now the whole world will know you are gifted.

Thank you, Wanza, "The Gospel Writer" Leftwich. That is who you truly are. Through your years of thinking you were barren, God filled you with purpose. Who would have thought our paths would cross; only God knew. Thank you for being a part of my life's journey. The book, "The Enemy in the Inner Me" has been shaped by the anointing God has blessed you with to publish. I will forever be grateful to you.

And thanks to you and you for reading this book and supporting the cause for cancer.

FOREWORD

We are fortunate to live in a society where its members have a right to life, liberty, and the pursuit of happiness. Constitutional, legislative, and municipal bodies safeguard the aforementioned privileges. Furthermore, violators who are found responsible for interrupting, invading, or impeding on the peace and good will of our society are enemies of that society and are subject to penalty imposed by the enforcers of society.

But what happens when the enemy is in the inner me? The Enemy in the Inner Me written by Theresa Hart presents a strategic battle plan to combat the devastating, dreadful, and in some cases deadly effects of cancer, the enemy of the body.

Theresa Hart has in this touching, tender, and tense exposé revealed the vast scope of consequences and challenges imposed on families, friends, and co-workers associated with loved ones victimized by this carnivorous disease.

Society is structured in a manner such that external enemies are eradicated through a clear set of rules. However, cancer, the internal enemy, cannot be as easily removed or destroyed. This harsh reality, concerning the unsympathetic nature of cancer is addressed with an honest tone, an uplifting construction, and a victorious resolve.

Theresa Hart has unveiled her innermost experience to help others suffering from cancer. Both therapeutic and informative, The Enemy in the Inner Me is a powerful read.

Bishop Eric R. Figueroa, Sr.,
Presiding Prelate

New Life Covenant Fellowship
Headquarters, Brooklyn, NY

Senior Pastor & Founder
New Life Tabernacle, Inc. Brooklyn, NY

INTRODUCTION

"I never thought it would happen to me."

I didn't think this would be my lot in life. We all have dreams and visions of what we would like our lives to be. Cancer was nowhere in my future or vision. It was not even a thought. I was always the kind of young girl that dreamed of having a wonderful family, beautiful children, and a handsome husband. God gave me all of it and more. I never asked for much; however, I nurtured what I was given to the best of my ability.

Cancer – the very word sends chills up and down my spine. Cancer is always associated with the word death. Cancer has claimed so many lives. I never thought I would be named in the number of men, women, families, and friends called survivors. Against all odds we have walked down the road called cancer and have defeated it in life and death. I have learned that it cannot take away our love, our dreams, our soul, and our spirit.

"I never thought it would happen to me." It did happen and it has made me appreciate life. I love with no strings attached and give because it's my reasonable service. I now wear this world as a loose garment. I'm not so attached that I can't see what life is really about.

When this title "The Enemy in the Inner me" was given to me by God, I thought it was going to be my trial sermon. Oh yes, God called me to the ministry to be an Evangelist. I was afraid of this calling because your life becomes an open book. Privacy is no longer an option. I asked, "Why did God call me?" I was not the worst of persons nor was I the best. Although I always loved working with and caring for people, I wasn't looking to become an Evangelist. This was something natural for me to do. I like being a positive influence.

Now I see why God gave me this title. It's so befitting. No one ever knows when their time of affliction or testing time in life will be. NOBODY knows they have cancer unless it is found by self exam or detected by healthcare professionals. That means it was hiding just like other diseases or situations we go through. The "Enemy in the Inner Me" exposes this disease for what it is.

An enemy is hiding in a place it doesn't belong in your body and in our world. God, give me the ability, the courage, and the boldness to tell this story of how cancer can change and transform the life of the one afflicted with cancer and everyone that is connected to them. There are some scary moments, some challenging moments, and a lot of happy moments. There are also some faithful moments when trusting in God is necessary. He's right there no matter what it looks like.

This is a story that most people won't tell. My story is up close and personal; it delves into the inner part of me. This disease has not only altered and disfigured my physical body, but it has changed me emotionally.

Through it all I have held on to my integrity and faith in God. Come with me through the corridors of my mind, body and spirit. Experience how the effects of this dreaded disease changed my life and the lives of so many others. This disease – the enemy of life – tried to destroy my life and my spirit. But I prevailed through faith and love.

CHAPTER ONE
THE DIAGNOSIS

I can remember exactly when I felt led to tell my story. In fact, it's very easy for me to remember. History was made that remarkable day in November. Barack Obama became the first black President of the United States of America. It was an historic day at its best for the nation and for me personally. It is the day that the spirit of the Lord led me to tell my story.

President Barack Obama started his journey as President and I began my journey through breast cancer. I heard there would be some good days and there would be some challenging days, but through it all, my faith could bring me through the testing times ahead; therefore, I did not complain because I already knew I had the victory!

Let's see... where should I start? How about at the beginning?

I was taking a shower one evening in June when I felt an oval shape on the left side of my left breast. I didn't think lump or cancer because I had just had a mammogram in May and the report came back that everything was fine. There is no history of cancer in my family so that was the furthest thing from my mind. To be honest, I just thought my breast was sore because my body was going through its monthly cycle.

I ignored it for about a week. When it didn't go away I called my doctor to set up an appointment. By then it felt like a swollen vein. I could hardly touch my left breast with my left arm. It was sensitive to the touch. I still did not think it was anything serious. I was following doctor's orders: When something is not right, check it out!

When he examined me, he sent me for a needle biopsy and a sonogram. The results came back benign. Of course they did; I was praying and believing God for the victory, but to tell the truth I was a little scared. This is the worst thing a woman wants to hear, "You have a lump in your breast" or "You have breast cancer".

The doctor explained to me that it was better out than in.

"What is better out than in?" I asked.

"Fibroadenomas are among the findings that were seen on your mammogram," he explained. "They are benign (not cancerous) breast tumors that are made of glandular and fibrous breast tissue."

He continued, "The atypical biopsy results do not really show that much activity. I suggest having it surgically removed."

I was relieved. This was a good report. I agreed to have the biopsy and the benign cyst removed.

Now, mind you, I recently made up my mind to go back to school to get my master's degree in social work at Adelphi University. I was scheduled to begin school the following month. I saw this as a minor inconvenience. I had the surgery and went home the same day.

I was glad it was over and that everything was benign and out of me.

Hallelujah!

Shortly after the surgery, I had a doctor's appointment for clearance to go back to work. My husband and I arrived on time for my appointment. The doctor called us into the office right away to meet with the surgeon.

I was waiting for him to tell me that everything was fine and I could go back to work. He did say that, in part, but then he said, "We found cancer behind the benign cyst."

Did he just say that?

He continued without a pause. "You have two choices: One is to have a lumpectomy, chemotherapy, and radiation, or have a mastectomy, chemotherapy, and radiation."

When he said "cancer" I went deaf.

I saw my life pass by me in a matter of seconds. I saw my children, my family members, and my friends. What had my life become so far? It's amazing how fast you can see your entire life pass before you.

The surgeon kept talking.

I blacked out in my mind. I heard him and I didn't hear him.

Cancer?

I saw his mouth moving, but I didn't hear what he was saying. My husband was confused and in a state of shock as I was.

"Wait a minute!" my husband exclaimed. "What do you mean my wife has cancer?" he asked.

"The cyst we found was benign. However, cancer was hiding behind the cyst."

He couldn't be telling the truth.

"The benign cyst was 2.0 cm and the cancer was 1.2 cm," the doctor continued.

Did he just quote size to me? It's cancer.

He kept talking. "I was surprised as well because there were no indications of cancer after all the tests that were done." He also stated that he removed it, but he would know for sure if he was successful once the pathology report comes back.

Could there be more?

He told us to set up an appointment to have an MRI done of my breast. I sat in a daze.

Motionless.

Speechless.

I didn't know whether to cry, scream or run out of his office. It took everything for me to hold back the tears. I couldn't believe this was happening.

I am a child of God. I serve God with all my heart. No, this can't be happening to me. God, haven't I already gone through enough physical challenges? Now this? Lord, I have had five surgeries in my life this one will make six and I'm not finished yet? Is this for real? Now I have to go through breast cancer. Please don't let this be. Please.

I sat there trying to be strong. I wanted to trust God through this process. I was scared to death and ready to run for my life. I wanted to get in my car and drive off into the sunset.

I prayed silently. *Lord, what are you doing to me?*

My husband and I walked out of the office as if nothing happened. We didn't want it to show on our faces that we received a bad report. We walked over to the receptionist area to set up an appointment for an MRI of my breast.

"It's going to be a while before you get an appointment," the receptionist stated. "You have to wait for authorization."

Was she kidding?

I couldn't stand there any longer. My knees began to buckle. My legs were about to betray me.

"I have to go sit in the car," I finally spoke.

The receptionist's eyebrows furrowed. Her eyes pleaded for me not to cry. The sting I felt in my eyes let me know that the tears were approaching. One more second and she would be picking me up off the floor.

I made it to the car in time to breakdown. I felt like a well of water was filling up inside me. It was ready to overflow. When I let it out, I felt some form of release. It enabled me to make it to the next second.

This was a one step process, I figured. I've never been here before. I did not know what to expect next. I was not sure how I was going to act or respond. I was in a place of uncertainty. I was trying to hold on to God's unchanging hand, but I felt like I was on a tightrope, trying to balance this diagnosis.

I wasn't doing a good job of it! I thought I was going to pass out under the pressure. I got myself together just enough to make some phone calls for comfort and support. The first person I called was my girlfriend, Marguerite who had gone through breast cancer the previous year.

Who would have thought that I would be making this phone call to her? She had chemotherapy treatments first to make sure all the cancer was gone. Then she had a mastectomy on her left breast. After the surgery she had radiation. I was with her the day before her operation. I spent the night with her in New Jersey.

We reminisced all night long about growing up together and how her breasts were so attractive that they got us into a lot of clubs in the past. Marguerite is a beautiful woman. When she was younger she was even more beautiful. Half Black and half Spanish, long hair, high cheekbones, a coke-bottle shape, and bowlegged. Oh my God, she was gorgeous!

We were laughing, joking and enjoying the moment. We had not seen each other in a couple of years. I'd wished we were seeing each other on other terms. We cleaned and straightened her place so she would be able to rest when she returned home from the surgery. Marguerite always had clothes and stuff all over the place.

I lived with Marguerite and her mother in my teenage days. It was challenging for my mother to care for her six children with minimum support from my father. So, whenever I could help make things easier for my mom, I did. Marguerite's mother said I could stay without a problem.

It's nice to be nice. I always tell that to my children. We laughed that night because we thought of ourselves as Oscar and Felix in *The Odd Couple*. Remember that show? Marguerite was like Oscar and I was like Felix. Who would have thought she would have to go through breast cancer.

I thank God I was there to support her. We got up the next morning and as we drove, we listened to Steve Harvey on the radio. He always starts out with giving God praise. This helped confirm our faith as we approached the hospital.

Now here I was calling her with this unexpected news. When I called her the tears were already coming down. I couldn't stop the tears. I was so afraid at that moment I couldn't even think. Marguerite answered the phone.

"I have breast cancer," my voice cracked.

"No, Terry!" She called me by my nickname. "Please, not you!" she pleaded. "I don't want anybody to go through what I had to go through. You are too good."

I explained to her what the doctor said.

"Get all your paperwork, reports, mammograms and sonograms together," Marguerite said. "Start looking for a breast cancer specialist."

That was the best advice she could have given me. Unfortunately, I was not comfortable with my current surgeon. I didn't know him. His bedside manner was awful. My husband didn't like him at all.

When we were at his office he explained my diagnosis to us with the door open. The nurse kept coming in. The phone kept ringing—and he answered it. As I sat in front of him, I tried to digest what he said to me, but with the door being opened, it seemed like the people could see inside. There was no privacy and no consideration for my privacy. I felt like the people in the waiting room knew what was going on. I felt so embarrassed. I don't know why, but I did.

My husband and I felt the doctor did not show any empathy. My family doctor referred me to him to do the biopsy because it had to be removed surgically. He was just supposed to remove the benign cyst, but behind it was the cancer and he took most of it out.

Now it was time for the next step. Everything was going so fast or it just seemed that way because of the nervousness and confusion I was battling within myself. Kevin was shaken up as well. We didn't know what to say to each other.

I tried to remember everything Marguerite told me to get from the doctor while I was at the office. My mind was so cloudy I couldn't think straight. The authorization took longer than I thought, so I stayed in the car while my husband went back in for me. I was not in any condition to deal with people.

The next person I called was my sister in the Lord and co-worker, Jamesetta.

"I have breast cancer," I said when she answered.

She didn't know what to say. She was just as disoriented as I was.

"Father God, in the Name of Jesus..." She started praying right then and there. I received the prayer because I knew, even though I was afraid, God would bring me through. I had to lean on Him like I never had before. I just kept hearing in my mind, "You have breast cancer".

Unbelievable.

I remembered scriptures in my head, but the fear was so overwhelming, I couldn't focus. My only release was to let the tears flow. I tried to keep myself and my mind busy. Being still was not a good thing for me. I had to keep talking it out. I had to talk to people who loved me.

I called my mother-in-law, Mrs. Hart.

"Mrs. Hart, the doctor said I have breast cancer."

"Oh, Terry!" I could hear the compassion in her voice. "We're just going to pray and believe God."

She reminded me that I haven't come all this way by faith for God to forget about me.

God, why me?

"I know," I responded to her.

As Mrs. Hart continued to console me, Kevin came out to the car.

"Let's go back into the doctor's office. They got the authorization for the MRI."

I got myself together the best I could. I looked strong on the outside, but felt like I was falling apart on the inside. My spirit was quoting scriptures.

"By His stripes I am healed..."

"All things work together for good to them who love God..."

"Trust in the Lord with all your heart..." God if this cup can pass; please let it. My emotions and feelings were so scattered that everything appeared to move like a fast movie scene.

All at once I started thinking about anyone that has ever received this kind of news.

"Oh my God, have mercy." The words escaped from my lips. You never really know what someone else is going through until you experience something similar.

CHAPTER TWO

Displaced, but Still Covered By God

After I received the approval for the MRI, we left. On the way home I called Bishop Matthew Johnson from St. Albans Deliverance. We were going to that church at the time. I told him the whole story. I explained the diagnosis I was given by the doctor. Bishop Johnson said that he would be praying for me and to keep him updated.

The Bible says to give honor to whom honor is due. I'd like to thank Bishop Matthew Johnson and the St. Albans Deliverance family for being there and praying for my family and me during a time that I was hurt, confused and angry.

Just like God prepared a whale for Jonah when he didn't want to go to Nineveh to minister to the people as God had instructed him, God prepared a safe-haven for my family and me while I was out of order.

1 Now the word of the LORD came unto Jonah the son of Amittai, saying,

2 Arise, go to Nineveh, that great city, and cry against it; for their wickedness is come up before me.

3 But Jonah rose up to flee unto Tarshish from the presence of the LORD, and went down to Joppa; and he found a ship going to Tarshish: so he paid the fare thereof, and went down into it, to go with them unto Tarshish from the presence of the LORD.

4 But the LORD sent out a great wind into the sea, and there was a mighty tempest in the sea, so that the ship was like to be broken.

5 Then the mariners were afraid, and cried every man unto his god, and cast forth the wares that were in the ship into the sea, to lighten it of them. But Jonah was gone down into the sides of the ship; and he lay, and was fast asleep.

6 So the shipmaster came to him, and said unto him, What meanest thou, O sleeper? arise, call upon thy God, if so be that God will think upon us, that we perish not.

7 And they said every one to his fellow, Come, and let us cast lots, that we may know for whose cause this evil is upon us. So they cast lots, and the lot fell upon Jonah.

8 Then said they unto him, Tell us, we pray thee, for whose cause this evil is upon us; What is thine occupation? and whence comest thou? what is thy country? and of what people art thou?

9 And he said unto them, I am an Hebrew; and I fear the LORD, the God of heaven, which hath made the sea and the dry land.

10 Then were the men exceedingly afraid, and said unto him. Why hast thou done this? For the men knew that he fled from the presence of the LORD, because he had told them.

11 Then said they unto him, What shall we do unto thee, that the sea may be calm unto us? for the sea wrought, and was tempestuous.

> 12 And he said unto them, Take me up, and cast me forth into the sea; so shall the sea be calm unto you: for I know that for my sake this great tempest is upon you.
>
> 13 Nevertheless the men rowed hard to bring it to the land; but they could not: for the sea wrought, and was tempestuous against them.
>
> 14 Wherefore they cried unto the LORD, and said, We beseech thee, O LORD, we beseech thee, let us not perish for this man's life, and lay not upon us innocent blood: for thou, O LORD, hast done as it pleased thee.
>
> 15 So they took up Jonah, and cast him forth into the sea: and the sea ceased from her raging.
>
> 16 Then the men feared the LORD exceedingly, and offered a sacrifice unto the LORD, and made vows.
>
> 17 Now the LORD had prepared a great fish to swallow up Jonah. And Jonah was in the belly of the fish three days and three nights.
>
> Jonah 1 (KJV)

I displaced my family because I was hurt. I thought it was God's plan and His strategy to move us. I was so wrong and so far from the truth.

I thank God for His covering, His grace, His mercy and His love that He blessed our family in spite of ourselves. My only regret is having separated from another family we had grown to love. It was a bitter-sweet separation. This time I was not hurt or confused.

I heard the Lord say to me, "It's time to go back home." It was clear that the Lord meant my home church.

I heard it for a year. I heard it through different messages. I hesitated because I wanted to make sure it was God this time and not me. Bishop Johnson and the St. Albans Deliverance Family were there for me and my family through one of the most challenging times in our lives. I was going through breast cancer and my mother had renal failure. Shortly after, while my husband and I were on vacation he ruptured his Achilles tendon.

There wasn't a time that Bishop Johnson and the St. Albans Deliverance Family ever stop praying for us. Nothing stopped Bishop Johnson from making countless visits to the hospital and nursing home to visit and pray with my mother; now that is the kind of love that goes from heart to heart and breast to breast.

During this time they saw what the transformation of this deadly disease called cancer did to my body. They saw me healthy and strong, then from weak to frail. They saw me vibrant and full of energy to no strength at all.

God had a place prepared for me. *Thank you, Lord, for being patient with me.*

It was a quiet ride home. The only thing my husband said was, "We are going to believe God and get a second opinion."

CHAPTER THREE
Telling the Family I Have Cancer

When I walked into the house my mother was standing at the top of the stairs.

"So, what did the doctor say?"

"Mommy, he said they found cancer in my breast."

My mother looked shocked. She was in disbelief and in denial just like I felt.

"Cancer is nowhere in our family," she stated. "Where did this come from? Just get another opinion to be one-hundred percent sure."

I went out to the store to be alone. I tried to process it all. When I returned home I prepared dinner and waited for my son to come home from school and my daughter to come home from work. I was really concerned about how they were going to take this news. I didn't want them to start crying and carrying on like I had a death sentence. In spite of everything, I knew I was going to be okay by faith.

Thoughts ran through my mind.

I don't believe this is happening to me.

Okay, don't lose it now. Girl, this is the time that you have to hold on to everything you know about God.

When the children came home I called them into my son's room and told them the diagnosis.

"I have breast cancer." *Did I just say that?*

"WHAT?" My son couldn't believe what I said.

My daughter looked the way I did earlier that day when the doctor gave me the news. Then she said, "You are going to be ALRIGHT!"

I was overwhelmed in my soul because we know God. Although the news was tough, we don't sorrow as others who have no hope in the Lord. I thank God for training up children in the way they should go in the Word of the Lord—so when they are old, when they are challenged, when they go through, they have confidence in whom they believe.

Thank you, Jesus.

At that moment I felt faith all around me from my family. A family that prays together stays together. It really does work.

That night I spoke to my brother, Prince.

"No, sis, stop playing!" When he realized it was real he was dismayed. I explained everything to him. I started feeling like a broken record.

I have breast cancer.

The cyst was benign, but cancer was behind it.

I have breast cancer.

I encouraged him and let him know that I was going to be alright. There I was still trying to be strong when I was ready to crumple. The next call I made was to my baby brother and sister-in-law.

I told Leveda and she was so sorry to hear it, but then said, "Terry, you know God; He did not bring you this far to leave you."

"I know," I said.

She did all she could to encourage me. She did a good job, but the facts remained. I was now dealing with breast cancer. I told her to tell my baby brother.

I couldn't talk about it anymore.

CHAPTER FOUR
Meeting the Right Doctors

I had to prepare for the next step; I had to find a breast cancer specialist. The next day I spoke to my girlfriend, Jamesetta about going into the hospital system and looking for a good breast cancer doctor. I thank God for a co-worker who is saved and a real Christian friend. I thank God that I was led by the Holy Spirit. When I called the hospital I got three referrals. I called the first one and left a message. I prayed every step of the way. This was serious. I wanted to be referred to the right doctor.

By the time I made the calls, Jamesetta, who I call "Prophetess" and she calls me "Bishop", (we just believe God for great and mighty things) called and said, "I was led to talk to one of my co-workers who just went through this process."

She went to her book and said, "Dr. Chen." She stated that her bedside manner was awesome. Then she asked another co-worker who was going through cancer about Dr. Chen. The co-worker replied, "She is a wonderful doctor."

I told Jamesetta that Dr. Chen was the third name on the list of referrals from the hospital. When I called Dr. Chen's office, I received such a wonderful and caring response. I felt comfortable speaking to the office manager. The manager told me that Dr. Chen was on vacation and that she would return after Labor Day.

I was surprised when Dr. Chen's office manager suggested that I get all of the films of my mammograms and sonograms for the last two years. In addition, I needed to get the pathology slide of the cancer and cyst that was removed and any other biopsy and reports that were done. Once I had everything she told me to—get this now—fax all reports so that she could email them to Dr. Chen to review while she was on vacation. If what she reviewed was urgent, Dr. Chen would have her assistant to see me; and if it could wait until she returned, she would call me back with an appointment ASAP!

It was so thoughtful and wonderful that the doctor cared that much that she would review my files even when she was on vacation. By that time, the other doctor's office called and left me a message. I did not return the call because I knew in my heart and spirit that Dr. Chen was the doctor for me.

I was captivated by Dr. Chen's office's response. I needed that kind of response to assure me and help me take the steps I needed to start this process and journey. Just for the record, make sure you find a doctor who is sensitive about your findings, whatever they may be. I started calling and making appointments to get all that was required. I told my doctor's office to fax all the reports necessary.

I made an appointment to get my mammogram and sonogram films and the pathology slide from the hospital where I'd had the surgery. I submitted everything that was required of me. Dr. Chen's office informed me that they received everything and would forward it to Dr. Chen. A week went by and it seemed like an eternity had passed. I had to wait it out by being patient, praying, trusting, and believing God. Isaiah 40:31 states, "But they that wait upon the LORD shall renew their strength; they shall mount up with wings as eagles; they shall run, and not be weary; and they shall walk, and not faint."

It was not an easy thing to do under the circumstances.

Hello... I have breast cancer; how long did I have to wait?

All kinds of things were going through my mind. *It can spread throughout my body. Will I live through this? Will I need to have my breast removed? Will I need chemo? Will my hair fall out?*

What torture I put myself through. They finally called and gave me an appointment for a week or so after I submitted the files. This was right after our 28th wedding anniversary.

This was really a hard pill to swallow. I wasn't going around telling people what I was going through. The only ones who knew were my family and my very close friends. Understand, I was taking baby steps every step of the way.

I still did not know what to expect from one minute to the next. I stayed busy so my own mind would not get the best of me. I realized going through this that I wasn't the only one affected by it.

My husband and children were really affected the most by this. People often do not realize that when you go through cancer, your family goes through it as well. They don't have the symptoms or have to take the therapy and medications, but the mental, emotional, and spiritual stress of processing what their loved one is going through is very difficult.

I know I keep saying it, but I could not believe that I was dealing with breast cancer; this was something that baffled my mind. The devil was talking to me. He told me things like I was going to die or that the doctor was going to remove my breast and on and on; he whispered in my ear like a recorder. I had to tune the devil out and concentrate on the word of God, my family, my friends, and all those who were encouraging me through all of this.

Finally, the day came for me to meet with Dr. Chen. We arrived at her office and went to the front desk. They greeted me with care and concern. We waited for about twenty minutes. Of course that seemed like forever.

They called my name and I said to myself, "Ok, girl, here you go!" My meeting with Dr. Chen was very pleasant, supporting, and reassuring. She closed her door and gave us privacy. The previous surgeon did not do this.

She introduced herself, and Kevin and I did the same.

"May I examine you?" Dr. Chen asked. I nodded. "Mr. Hart, will you wait in the waiting room until I am finished?"

Kevin obliged and exited the office.

Dr. Chen examined my breast. "The incision is great," she said. "I'm going into the same incision and take out the cancer cells that remain."

I got dressed and went back into her office. We called for Kevin join us.

"I've read the reports. I don't think you need to have a mastectomy."

I wanted to shout, scream, leap for joy right there, but my spirit did all that.

Dr. Chen continued, "The cancer is 1.2 centimeters and it is isolated. There is no sign that it has spread."

I gave God another praise right there.

"There are some specks in the area." Dr. Chen explained that she would go in and scoop out a large amount around the margin where the cancer cells were showing. Also, she would test three of my lymph nodes to make sure they were not infected. If they were infected, she was going to remove them as she did the lumpectomy.

She was very informative. Dr. Chen continued to clarify everything for me and Kevin. She defined in detail what a lumpectomy and mastectomy were and gave us the information to walk away with. It was a lot of information to contain at one time. Based on my medical reports, all the films and slides, it wasn't as bad as it appeared.

"Thank you, Jesus!" *Did I say that aloud? It's okay.*

Dr. Chen was so hospitable that my husband and I were very happy and pleased with her. She scheduled the lumpectomy surgery, but I had to go for an MRI of the breast. I was not looking forward to that. I don't like being in closed-in areas or spaces.

The day of the MRI I prayed, "Lord, please help me through this. Don't let me panic and go through anxiety disorder."

I had the nicest technician, who was very patient and calm with me. I tell you when you know God, He will put people in your way to help guide, support, instruct, nurture and encourage you in whatever it is you must go through.

The technician said, "You are going to hear a lot of noise, but don't be alarmed."

"Okay…and don't pay me any attention either because I am going to be praying out loud." I meant that. I really did.

He started the MRI machine and I started to pray. Before I knew it the test was over. It wasn't as bad as I thought. I was positioned to enter the MRI machine feet first, lying on my stomach. Then I put my breasts into two cup holes. The top of the table had a big circle opening for my face. My arms and hands rested in an oval position on brackets. I couldn't see anything. *Thank God.* I would have lost my mind if I'd had to go in lying on my back. That reminds me of a coffin and that would not have worked.

CHAPTER FIVE
The Call of Reconciliation

I began to reflect on my life and the diagnosis of breast cancer. It made me think about the people that I love with all my heart. This led my mind to Bishop Eric R. Figueroa, Sr., my Bishop for over twenty years. I caused my family to leave our home church over something that I don't even remember now. This clearly means that it was not crucial. What I have learned through this whole growth and development process is, "never make any decisions when you are mad, hurt or confused." Stop, step back, calm down, breathe, and pray, then wait for an answer.

I called Bishop Eric R. Figueroa, Sr. because he did not know what I was going through. I called him with tears in my eyes, yearning to hear his voice.

"I believe God," Bishop stated the New Life Tabernacle Church motto when he answered.

"I believe God," I responded. "Praise the Lord, Bishop."

He immediately said, "Tee." He knew my voice right away. That is a father.

"Bishop."

"Is everything ok?" he asked. As if he knew something wasn't right.

"The doctor said I have beast cancer."

"Oh, Theresa, I'm so sorry," Bishop said.

I explained to him that they found it and that I needed surgery. When I finished, he prayed and I cried. To hear his voice and to feel the love through the phone while he prayed for me made me so sorry that I wasn't where I needed to be.

After he finished praying, he said, "Keep me posted, Tee." We ended with, "I love you."

It was so wonderful that I can't explain it well enough. When love is real, it really does cover a multitude of sins! After the phone call with Bishop Figueroa and the prayer, I had the strength to go through the next step in the process.

CHAPTER SIX
Preparing for Surgery

The week before surgery, I sat at my desk at work trying to act normal. I tried to do business as usual, but on the inside I felt like I was on a roller coaster ride. I don't like roller coasters at all. The first and last time I was on a rollercoaster I was sixteen years old. I got a little ulcer from being scared half to death!

I must say that I have the best co-workers in the world. They rallied around me in such a way that the love and support lifted the nervousness right off of me.

Everything began to move fast. I took care of all of my paperwork at work for disability. I set up my work for coverage and things at home because I knew after the surgery I would not be able to do anything but rest and heal. My family and I thoroughly cleaned my bedroom.

Jamesetta and I went to Macy's and bought a beautiful bed-in-the-bag set and nice scented candles.

"You will be spending a lot of time in here so make it pleasant. You want to feel comfortable and relaxed," she said. "You don't want to look around and see things that need to be done." I am a neat freak anyway, so it was right up my alley to clean. Also, it took my mind off of what was going to happen the next day.

The night before the surgery, my bedroom was nice, fresh, pretty, and smelling beautiful. My husband and I woke up the next morning prayed up, refreshed and ready to go through this journey together. I was so pleased that my mother-in-law took off work and willingly came to be there with us.

This is the sixth surgery. God what is going on? Haven't I been through enough physically? Is this my fate, too?

The voice in my head continued to ask, "Why me?"

We arrived at the hospital's Pre-surgical department. I don't know why, but I felt ashamed and naked. Maybe it was because it was the same hospital I worked in. I was thinking that everybody would know my business. I prayed that I wouldn't see anybody! This way I would not have to explain or lie. Honestly, I did not want everybody in my business.

The nurse called me and my family in the back to do the paperwork. I must tell this part of the story. After filling out all of the forms, we were told to go to the waiting room.

"You will be called in the back when they are ready to prepare you for the surgery," the hospital worker said.

I thank God for my mother-in-law. She fasted and prayed the entire time. I thank God for praying people around me. I also thank God for my husband; other than God, he was the closest one to me and he did not shy away from this challenge.

While I sat in the waiting room, I felt my Bishop Figueroa in my spirit. I went to the bathroom and called him.

"Bishop, I'm getting ready to have the surgery."

He prayed with me. "Call me or have your family call me after the surgery. Love you, Tee."

"Love you, too, Bishop." I hung up the phone and returned to the waiting area.

"Theresa Hart." They called my name. We went back to where they prepare the patients for surgery. The nurse showed me where to go. The nurse gave me a gown to put on and my mother-in-law helped me get undressed. My husband put everything in the hospital bag.

I can't believe I am having surgery again.

The nurse set up the IV. The anesthesiologist explained everything to me. Dr. Chen came in and drew on the area of my left breast, the area where she would operate.

"When you take me into the operating room, do not lay me flat on my back until I'm sedated." I had to tell them that. Don't ask. It's a paranoia thing.

Kevin, Mrs. Hart, and I were talking to pass the time and to keep our minds off of what was about to happen. Thankfully, my co-worker, Maggie came to show her support. It was thoughtful, but that's just how Maggie is. We talked until they came and said that they were ready for me.

My stomach felt like it dropped into my lap, but it was time to do this.

"See you later," I said.

Maggie returned to the office.

"Okay, God, here we go!" I said as they wheeled me in the operating room.

"I just saw your sister," Dr. Chen stated.

I had a stupid look on my face until I realized who she was talking about. Jamesetta! I had looked for Jamesetta, but unbeknownst to me, she was in the back speaking to Dr. Chen regarding me. She let Dr. Chen know that she came highly recommended because she was referred by two co-workers. Dr. Chen assured Jamesetta that everything was going to be fine. I'm thankful for true friendships with people who have your best interest at heart.

The surgery was a success. I pulled through it with God on my side. As I waited in the recovery room for the anesthesia to wear off, I woke up feeling very cold. Of course the first thing I did was feel my breast.

I started feeling everything that was done. The pain medicine was wearing off. I signaled for the nurse to let her know that I was in pain. My left side by my left breast felt tight and drawn together in the area by the breast. I guess it was a good thing to feel what I felt; it let me know that it was a job well done.

I felt left-sided. She gave me two Percocets to attack the pain. They gave me some juice and crackers and prepared me for the discharge summary. By that time my husband and mother-in-law came in the recovery area. I assured them that I was fine. I wanted to get out of the hospital and go home and get in my bed.

My husband and my mother-in-law helped me get dressed.

"She's almost ready to go to the car," the nurse said.

The nurse gave me the discharge papers and a prescription for Percocet.

"Mrs. Hart, call Dr. Chen's office to make an appointment in two weeks," the nurse instructed.

I could not wait to get out of the hospital. I wanted to go home to my place of serenity; in my comfortable bedroom that was prepared for me to rest while I went through this process.

Chapter Seven

Recovery

The next day I called and made my appointment with Dr. Chen. Two weeks seemed liked two years. I took those two weeks to relax and heal. I enjoyed my family taking care of me because I am always caring or doing for someone else. I was a good patient.

The day of the appointment I was excited and nervous at the same time. It was the unveiling of how the incision looked. I was eager to hear her good report. I believed God for the VICTORY! It was pleasant meeting with her because her compassion for what she does was evident.

She loves what she does. She genuinely cares for each patient.

Dr. Chen told me she removed the remaining cancer cells that were in the margin area of where the cancer was (in the left breast on the left side of the breast). I had three weeks to heal and prepare for radiation, so I thought. The doctor stated I probably would not need chemotherapy because my situation was different.

The cancer was isolated, but she wanted me to make an appointment with the Radiologist and the Oncologist. The three weeks passed and I felt good about everything. I thought that I would not need to have chemotherapy.

First I went to see the Radiologist. Dr. Lim was a sweetheart. God really did put doctors in my life that were a blessing to me in more ways than one. The whole radiation process was incredible and scary at the same time. Dr. Lim explained an upper body cast would be created just for me because I would have to be positioned in it the same way every time I came for radiation.

She informed me that I would be tattooed. I got scared.

What kind of tattoo? I don't believe in any of that.

The doctor saw the concern on my face.

"There will be pin dots placed around the left breast so the radiation machine will calculate and know where to zoom in for the radiation treatment," she explained.

This was very serious and a delicate procedure. The treatment would take place by my heart; the dimensions had to be precise. I was positioned and a body cast was molded on me. It was similar to how they make a cast when you break your arm or leg. My whole upper left side had to be sculpted.

I really felt like I was the clay and the doctor was the potter with a diagram of my own specifications. Every time I came (36 treatments), I would have to lay in the cast and be positioned. When the machine calculated the measurements, it zoomed in and filled my breast with radiation.

Amazing!

"You will experience tenderness, some skin burning, pigmentation of the skin, heaviness in your left breast and sensitivity," the doctor said. "The radiation builds up in the area where the cancer is concentrated. Your left breast will be bigger than your right breast."

"Great! I will look even more like a freak!" *This was getting better and better!*

I wanted to start the radiation and get it over with.

CHAPTER EIGHT
The shock of my life!

I kept thinking that I would not need chemotherapy.

So I thought!

Within the next two weeks I met with the Director of Oncology regarding chemotherapy.

"Do you want me to come with you?" Kevin asked.

"No," I said confidently. "They are just going to explain chemo as an option." I was so hell bent on not needing chemo that I didn't think I needed any support.

I thought they were going to say, "Mrs. Hart, you don't need chemotherapy…make an appointment with the radiologist."

That didn't happen. I met with the oncologist and his assistant. They were both very nice. The oncologist explained my condition in depth to me.

"You are negative across the board," he began. "This is good. You don't carry the HER2 gene, which is another plus." Then it took a turn.

"Because of the size of the cancer, you will need to have four treatments of the chemotherapy."

My heart felt like it was going to fall right out of my chest. My hope and faith suddenly plunged. At that moment I felt hopeless. I fell apart and cried. I was not prepared for this decision and not prepared to deal with this alone. The doctor and his assistant saw the state of shock on my face.

"Why didn't you bring your husband?" the doctor asked.

"I didn't think I was going to need chemotherapy." I shook my head.

Before I could start the chemotherapy, I had to complete a series of tests. This meant I had to go through several different machines. The first one was a full body bone scan, then a head and chest CT scan, also called a CAT scan. The last test would be a pelvic and abdominal CAT scan. I was so afraid. As I mentioned earlier, I do not like closed in spaces.

I prayed that these machines were not closed in. I left the oncologist's office very upset and afraid. I questioned my faith. The only thing I could think about was the side effects of chemotherapy. The more I thought about my hair falling out, my nails turning black and having the "cancer look", I grew more filled with dread. God knows what else could happen to my body. I pulled the car over and cried.

I felt so, so, alone. I didn't even feel God. How could I be strong against something I was so afraid of? Amazingly, I could be strong for my family and everybody else, but when it came to me, I fell apart. I thought about who I could call and talk to.

I called my prayer partner, Jamesetta.

"I have to have chemotherapy," I said.

She couldn't believe it either. So much was going through my mind that I had to literally grab a thought and hold on to it. My mind raced so much. It reflected on Joyce Meyers' book, *Do It Afraid.* I needed that at that time. The process of breast cancer from surgery to recovery can, indeed, be overwhelming. I faced the fact that I was petrified.

I called Kevin and explained to him that I would need chemotherapy treatments. I heard the surprise in his voice. Being the wonderful husband that he is, he did everything in his power to encourage me when he needed encouragement, himself. I informed him of the tests I had to have done by my next appointment. The oncologist wanted him to accompany me. Based on my first shocking visit, I needed a support system in place. This was definitely a process where I didn't need to be alone.

I thought about all the cancer survivors along with other devastating diseases many people have to deal with by themselves. What heroic testimonies.

I also called Marguerite. She was in shock. She understood what I was about to go through and she loved me so much she didn't want to see me go down that road. Marguerite prayed for me for the first time right on the phone. I was so moved and touched by her sincerity to pray for me that I began to cry and praise God. It was an on-time prayer. It seemed as if I was losing the battle.

I was trying to be strong, but it was not working. Sitting in my car outside of my job, I felt so alone. I knew God was there, I knew the Holy Spirit was present, I knew the angels were all around me, but at that moment I could not see or feel anything but my hurt and my pain. I don't understand how anybody could go through something so devastating and not know God; it's too much for one person to grasp. You will crumble under the pressure and the weight of a thing or situation that is bigger than you. That's why you need to know a BIG GOD that can be touched with the feelings of our infirmities.

When you know God for yourself, it is an amazing experience, regardless of the fact that you are going through a challenging situation. You can make it through. It's just like when you get in trouble or a hurting child calls out to their parents, our heavenly Father is right there waiting for you to reach out to Him.

In spite of all I knew about the Lord, I was having this emotional battle on the inside accepting the fact that I had breast cancer. The feeling of embarrassment crept up on me again. I guess I wasn't ready to share what I was going through with anybody that was not close to me.

Every time I went to the Oncology building, it was as if my life was an open book because I worked for the hospital. There was no telling who I might run into. What would I say and how would my reaction be with them? Crazy!

Sometimes I would see some of my co-workers, but they wouldn't see me. I looked hard to make sure that no one saw me going in that building, especially in the state I was in.

HELP, Lord!

One minute my life consisted of working, family, church, community outreach, going out and enjoying life, then the next minute, I was being inundated with doctors' visits and testing. This was really dealing with "the battle of the mind".

Feelings I never felt before were all of a sudden taking me on an emotional rollercoaster. Most of my tests were done at a diagnostic imaging center, so much so that it seemed as if all the employees knew why I was there. I believed that was the devil trying to distract me. I continued to pray and trust God even though I did not understand everything I was going through.

CHAPTER NINE
A Praise Break!

Let me put in a praise right here!

I thank my Lord and Savior Jesus Christ for loving me. He allowed me to become a Christian and live this Kingdom life. Even though I am going through breast cancer and it appears that my whole world has been shaken, I still give God all the glory and honor. I don't know the whys or the ultimate reason behind this; however, I know I can do all things through Christ which gives me strength; whether I feel it or not.

2 Corinthians 4:7-10 states "But we have this treasure in earthen vessels, that the excellency of the power may be of God, and not of us. We are troubled on every side, yet not distressed; we are perplexed, but not in despair; Persecuted, but not forsaken; cast down, but not destroyed; Always bearing about in the body the dying

of the Lord Jesus that the life also of Jesus might be made manifest in our body."

These scriptures gave me a level of trust and hope in God that I didn't have before. I've never been here before, so I reached down deep and looked up to my heavenly Father from whom I can draw strength. I'm confident in knowing that no matter how bad my situation looks, there is always someone that is doing worse than me.

John 3:16 states "For God so loved the world that he gave His only begotten Son that whosoever believeth on Him will not perish but have everlasting life." Having a relationship with God is key in getting through any tough situation. Accept Him [GOD] and you will feel what I am feeling right now. Just believe that the Lord Jesus Christ died on the cross for your sins and receive Him into your heart. See…don't you feel His love? I know you do. God Bless you. He will work everything out.

CHAPTER TEN
I'm His Wife

"To live is so startling it leaves little time for anything else." This quote by Emily Dickinson touched my life. In spite of everything, I knew that I wanted to live.

I WANT TO LIVE!

Two weeks passed and all my test results were in. It was time for my husband and me to meet with the oncologist. The doctor explained to my husband that I needed chemotherapy.

My husband stopped the doctor dead in his tracks and asked him to explain it to him so that he could understand. Kevin made a statement that let it be known that his confidence and this situation were in God's hands. Then he said,

"This is my wife and I love her very much. I want the best for my wife. I want her around for a long time, so speak to me where I can understand my role as her husband and caregiver during this challenging time."

The doctor and the nurse practitioner were pleased to see his care, love, and concern for me. This caused the doctor to explain the procedure in a way that gave us a better understanding of the entire process.

CHAPTER ELEVEN
Preparing for Chemotherapy

I was scheduled to start chemotherapy in early November. The nurse practitioner took me to the second floor where I would be administered chemotherapy. I made the appointment. Then one of the nurses showed me around. I was so extremely uncomfortable.

The nurse checked my veins on my right arm to see if they would be able to withstand the four chemo treatments.

“If your veins can’t, we will give you a port,” The nurse practitioner stated.

At the same time, I learned that I could no longer have blood drawn or have my blood pressure taken or anything done on my left arm because the cancer was found on the left side. As I left, I realized that this was the department I would normally walk through when I would take the shortcut through to another department.

WOW! Who would have thought that I would be here – not taking the shortcut, but as a patient. I met Kevin outside at the car. It was all we could do to process what we'd just heard.

Chemotherapy?

Can they use my veins or will they have to give me a port?

Kevin looked at me and said, "We will leave everything in God's hands."

The chemotherapy was less than a week away and that's all I could think about. I prayed and read the word of God to encourage myself. The Spirit of the Lord led me to Philippians 4:8, "Finally, brethren, whatsoever things are true, whatsoever things are honest, whatsoever things are just, whatsoever things are pure, whatsoever things are lovely, whatsoever things are of good report; if there be any virtue, and if there be any praise, think on these things." This scripture encouraged me to think on the goodness of God and stop dwelling on the negative.

I also read Ephesians 6: 10-18.

> 10 Finally, my brethren, be strong in the Lord, and in the power of his might.
>
> 11 Put on the whole armor of God that ye may be able to stand against the wiles of the devil.
>
> 12 For we wrestle not against flesh and blood, but against principalities, against powers, against the rulers of the darkness of this world, against spiritual wickedness in high places.
>
> 13 Wherefore take unto you the whole armor of God that ye may be able to withstand in the evil day, and having done all, to stand.

14 Stand therefore, having your loins girt about with truth, and having on the breastplate of righteousness;
15 And your feet shod with the preparation of the gospel of peace;
16 Above all, taking the shield of faith, wherewith ye shall be able to quench all the fiery darts of the wicked.
17 And take the helmet of salvation, and the sword of the Spirit, which is the word of God:
18 Praying always with all prayer and supplication in the Spirit, and watching thereunto with all perseverance and supplication for all saints;"

I had to build up my faith and get myself ready for this unplanned and unrehearsed script that I was handed at this time in my life.

CHAPTER TWELVE
An Unexpected Change

"You need emergency surgery," the doctor said. "The CAT Scan we took of the lower abdominal area shows that you have a cyst on your ovary. I don't believe it's cancer. However, before you start chemotherapy, we must take care of it."

Did he say emergency surgery? What in the world?

I couldn't think. I went blank!

I felt the fear. I listened to him in fear. I could not think of anything else to do. It felt like I was in the twilight zone. Wasn't I dealing with enough? Did I really need another surgery to remove a cyst that could be cancerous?

What is happening to me?

My oncologist set up an emergency appointment for me to meet with an OB/GYN Oncologist that specializes in ovarian cancer. I wrote all the information down even though my mind was in a fog. First thing in the morning I had to meet with this doctor.

When I got off the phone, it appeared as if I was doing everything in slow motion. I was trying to hold it together, but in actuality I was falling apart. My hand went numb from holding the phone so tightly. I was still recovering from the lumpectomy surgery, preparing to start chemotherapy and now this – a cyst.

I did not look forward to telling my family disappointing news again. I told my husband, son and daughter about this unexpected surgery. Their reactions mimicked my own—blank stares of fear and uncertainty.

Lord, what is going on?

Everyone did their best to comfort me. I went upstairs and told my mother; again, a blank stare. Needless to say I was frightened. I know what it feels like when fear consumes you. Even though it felt like the enemy was getting the best of me, in my soul I knew that for some reason, God was allowing this to happen.

Don't ask me to explain it. I just knew that this was something God was going to use to get the glory out of my life! I began to prepare myself to go in this new direction. The oncologist apologized for this unexpected news. He hoped it was nothing so that we could continue with the chemotherapy as planned.

I pondered the doctor's statement. "If the cyst is cancerous, we will have to approach the chemotherapy from a different perspective." He said he would have to consider treatment for both breast and ovarian cancer.

I didn't want to hear that at all. At that moment, I thought about the thousands of people who received this kind of phone call and the news wasn't good. My prayer is that God would bless you! Be encouraged, God will bring you through this and bless your life at the same time. I don't know why we go through certain things in life, but at the end there is victory when you have God on your side.

At the time, I honestly struggled to see my own victory. My faith and trust were in there somewhere. I just couldn't find it through the fear. I thought about the saying, "Don't let the devil see you sweat." At the moment, this was an understatement.

CHAPTER THIRTEEN

Preparing for the Second Surgery

The next morning, I woke up in a daze. Did I dream it all? I thought, *Any second now, I'm going to realize it was all a dream and my life will be back to normal.*

NOT!

I couldn't even cry and that's not normal for me. Crying is therapy; when you can't talk about it, you can cry it out. That was not even working. This was a whole lot to swallow.

I didn't know what to expect. I didn't know what God was allowing and I sure didn't know how to handle any of it. I got dressed and was out the door early in the morning, heading to a doctor's office that I didn't know anything about.

We got there and waited for what seemed like a lifetime to me. When I heard my name called, my heart skipped a beat. I leaped from the chair. As we walked through the hallway, the nurse turned to me and said, "Don't worry. You are going to be fine."

Did fear show on my face?

The doctor came in the office. She was nice but straight to the point. She had to examine me. This released my husband for a few moments. He went back to the waiting area. He was glad to go for a few minutes. This was a lot for him to process, as well. Kevin dealt with this in his own way.

The doctor had my paperwork because my oncologist had faxed everything over the night before. They were not playing. The urgency of everything scared me. I explained to the doctor that I'd had a hysterectomy in 1999 due to a fibroid in my uterus. My OB/GYN doctor left one of my ovaries so it wouldn't knock me into menopause early. This doctor stated that whatever was left she would take out. "If I find cancer," she said, "you will have to have chemotherapy for breast and ovarian cancer.

Was she serious? Lord, I need you, now!

The doctor scheduled the surgery for a few days later.

"If all goes well, the healing process will take about four weeks. You will be able to start chemotherapy shortly thereafter."

I'm happy to report that the surgery was successful. The cyst was not malignant, thank God! However, my whole body hurt. I had two surgeries within eight weeks. My body yelled at me from the inside saying, "What are you doing to me?" I replied to myself, "I wish I could answer you, I'm speechless."

I just wanted to go home and get in my bed. I had prepared my room to be comfortable; I knew that I would be in it a while; I did not know I would be in there longer than expected!

I was grateful for the doctor. Although my regular OB/GYN is very good; this doctor was good as well and she was also closer to my home than my current OB/GYN doctor. I wanted her to be my doctor. The doctor quickly corrected me. She said, “You don’t want me to be your doctor. I only deal with women who have cancer.” I gladly got the hint. My follow-up visit with her was my last. I thanked God that I had the victory. So, I thought.

Almost two weeks after the surgery I was healing well. I was on schedule to start chemotherapy in nearly two weeks. It was a Friday night and my husband ordered pizza. I love pizza. I had a small slice because I still was not prepared to eat a full meal. I ate several small meals instead of the normal three large meals.

That night as I got ready for bed my stomach felt a little upset. I thought it was because of the surgery. I took a pain pill and laid down, thinking that I had overdone it during the day. As the evening wore on I wasn’t feeling any better, and at about two in the morning the pain woke me up. I tried to stay quiet and not alarm anybody, but by seven o’clock in the morning I realized something wasn’t right.

I took more pain medicine trying to numb the pain; I made myself vomit and I drank water to try and flush it out of my system. I tried everything. I prayed that I would not open the wound where I was stitched. I suffered all night thinking the pain would pass, but it didn't.

On Saturday morning I was in so much pain; I didn't know what was going on. The pain felt worse than labor pains and I didn't think that was possible. My husband was cooking breakfast as he always does on Saturday morning. By then I was almost under the bed clutching on the bed comforter pulling it down and using it as support like a pillow. I screamed, which really alarmed everybody in the house. I had already called 911. When my family came in the room I told them I had called 911 because I couldn't take the pain anymore.

I got dressed the best I could. Right before the ambulance got there, the pain hit me so hard I almost went under the bed. When the Emergency Medical Service workers got there, they took me out screaming like I was a crazy woman; and for a moment I thought I had lost it.

I could not figure out what was going on. That was the worst ride ever in the ambulance. They strapped me down. I continued to scream. It felt as if they weren't paying me any attention. I know that wasn't really true because that ambulance was moving very fast. By the time I got to the hospital, I did not care what I looked like. They sat me in the hallway of the ER right across from the nurses' station. It appeared as if I wasn't important. Then I really I started acting like I was crazy because it seemed like they were taking their time. I know it wasn't like that, but I was in excruciating pain.

Finally, they took me in a room, put me in a bed and hooked me up to an IV so they could give me morphine. When the morphine hit my system the pain subsided enough for the doctors to talk to me to find out what happened. I explained that I had surgery three weeks prior and that I was fine until I had a slice of pizza the night before.

They sent me to have a CAT scan of the abdominal area. When the test results came back, the doctor stated, “You have a bowel obstruction.”

“What is a bowel obstruction?” I asked.

“A bowel obstruction is the condition that occurs when a section of the bowel, small or the large intestine becomes totally or partially blocked, so that stool cannot pass through it.”

I still didn’t get it. The doctor stated, “Everything is moving around in your body because of the surgery and it is getting itself back in order. It is possible that by eating the pizza, which takes a lot to digest because of the cheese, that it could have aided in the bowel obstruction.”

I looked at him with disbelief. The doctor admitted me for observation. I asked the doctor if he got in touch with the doctor who did the surgery. He told me he was waiting to hear back from her. Originally, I told the EMS workers to take me to LIJ where I had the surgery, but they explained to me that they had to take me to the closest hospital. I was in too much pain to dispute.

They took me to my room. By the time I reached the room my husband, daughter, and girlfriend, Jamesetta were there to give support. Unfortunately, my roommate was a very disorderly and confused patient. My family also complained about the patient in my room. I was really trying to ignore her. Then a blessing came my way. The doctor came in and told me I was being transported to the hospital where I'd had the surgery.

I was so glad to leave that room. I began to thank God. I arrived at the other hospital around eleven o'clock in the evening. Everything was prepared for me as if I was someone special. *I am!* I was the only one in the room. The bed was by the window. It allowed me to see outside and look at the stars in the sky. It was quiet and so peaceful. My family and friend commented that the Lord prepared a place of rest for me. I was so thankful to be in a familiar place.

The nurse came in and continued to give me the morphine in small doses because my doctor didn't want my body to suffer. I was scheduled to see her in the morning. My family and friend, Jamesetta were so content that I was comfortable; they were able to leave and be at peace because I was able to rest comfortably. I said goodnight to them and went right to sleep.

I had barely slept the night before. My body was drained and exhausted. As I drifted off to sleep, I wondered how much more this body of mine would be able to take.

The next morning I felt like I ran into a wall. My body was so sore as if I was in a physical fight. In a way I was. There was a battle going on on the inside of me. I saw the OB/GYN Oncologist and she explained to me the same thing the ER doctor said in regards to the bowel obstruction.

"I'm going to take you off morphine and give you another kind of medication to help relax your bowels," she said. "I also don't want to open you back up in order to help you move your bowels.

Of course, I didn't want that either!

The same day, my oncologist came to see me.

"Theresa what is going on with you?" he asked. "Your body doesn't want to act right, I see."

"Tell me about it." I responded.

"You are a week away from treatment. You have to be strong enough for your chemotherapy or it will be pushed back."

I really didn't want to hear that. Truth was, I didn't want the chemotherapy treatments, but I didn't want to prolong the process either.

I rested for almost a week so my body could get back to functioning normally and have a regular bowel movement without any complications. This was the week I should have been home resting, but I found myself back in the hospital before the chemotherapy treatments.

I enjoyed the stay because I got a chance to see some of my co-workers who I liked a great deal. I spend almost more time at work than I do at home. I have a job family that I enjoy seeing, working with, talking and praying with, and doing so many other things with them. We celebrate birthdays, our children's successes, and we genuinely care for each other. You don't always find that on a job. After four days, I went home to prepare for chemotherapy the following week.

I realized that I went from one condition to another, but God saw me through, step by step.

CHAPTER FOURTEEN
Chemotherapy

I will never forget my first day of chemotherapy treatment. I prayed on my way to the hospital. I prayed for strength to endure. Thoughts rushed through my mind, but I continued to pray.

I don't believe that I am going through this.

I have breast cancer?

Unbelievable!

I prayed I didn't see anybody I knew, as well. I went by myself. Why? I guess I needed to do it by myself. Did I have anything to prove? No. But there are just some things in life only you and God can go through.

My husband and daughter were so awesome in driving me around all the time. Their jobs and bosses were very supportive. I thank God for favor. I pulled up to the hospital building. They had already given me a pass to park in the parking lot every time I came. The parking attendant was very nice.

I needed for everybody and every step I took on that day to be nice. I arrived at the second floor, went to the reception desk and gave my name. Approximately fifteen minutes later, the nurse called me. She escorted me to the cubicles in the back. Each one had a television, a nice reclining chair, a desk where you can plug up your laptop, or your preference of electronic items that you may have.

For the first treatment they sit you close to the nurses' station so if there are any reactions they will be able to monitor you and address the matter at hand quickly. I sat down in the chair. They gave me a pillow to put behind my head.

"Would you like to look at TV?" the nurse asked.

"No, thank you. I have my portable DVD player."

As the chemotherapy went in, I wanted to listen to the word of God that cleanses and heals. By listening to the word of God, I knew that God would give me the confidence that I needed to get through this surprising journey. I had to listen to something spiritual and uplifting.

As they prepared the IV, I prayed within myself. My veins are not that great and I did not want a port. It is a four-hour process. Two hours each for each medicine. Taxotere and Cytoxan are two of the strongest chemotherapy medications. I braced myself for the pain.

"Relax, Theresa," the nurse said.

I took a deep breath. The needle went in without a problem. They gave me some type of liquid to keep the nutrients in my body. Twenty minutes later they gave me the first medicine, Taxotere. I felt the medicine go in my vein. A cool feeling went up my arm.

I put the earplugs in my ears and began to listen to the preached word. As soon as the medicine hit my system I had a reaction. I turned to the nurse, without panicking.

"I can't breathe," I said softly.

In less than one second I had five people around me. I gasped for air. My heart raced. The nurse stopped the medication and gave me a shot of Benadryl in my veins. In a matter of seconds I started breathing normally.

"How do you feel?" the doctor asked. "It's ok, you will be fine. Do you feel dizzy?"

"I'm OK," I answered. "I'm fine now." Once the Benadryl went through my system it was as if nothing happened. The doctor explained that each person reacts differently to the medication. They didn't want to give me the Benadryl first because they wanted to see what kind of reaction I would have. They continued with Taxotere.

Two hours later, the nurse started me on Cytoxan. I listened to some of my CDs and slept off and on. When I finished the treatment, I felt pretty good; they gave me steroids as well. I was ready to do a lot the next day, but the doctor asked me to come in and get a booster shot for the marrow in my bones. Apparently, the chemotherapy treatments eat the marrow in your bones.

"It's best to get this shot so that your bones remain strong," the nurse stated.

The next day, I went in for the shot. They gave the shot in my hip. It hurt like crazy! Afterward, my daughter and I went shopping. By the end of the day I started to feel everything that had happened over the past two days.

I needed to go home and get in my bed. By the time Sunday came I felt like a bulldozer had run over me. Better yet, I felt like I was 90 years old. Everything on and in my body hurt. They told me that in about two to three days I would begin feeling pain, discomfort, and maybe sick to my stomach. They were not lying. I felt all of the above. I didn't know I could feel so awful.

I got this taste in my mouth that tasted like metal or sulfur; the foods tasted the same way, as well. I lost my appetite and desire for food. Food that I loved, I now hated. Food I didn't really care for I ate. I had more of an appetite for food with salt than sweets.

It was a rule of thumb that you should eat small meals versus your basic three square meals a day while going through this process. It seemed the fuller you were, the sicker you became. The last thing the doctors wanted was for me to vomit and stress my body more than necessary.

The booster shot caused the marrow in my bones to multiply too much, which caused my bones to ache something awful. I could hardly walk. I didn't say anything or call the doctor because I thought it was part of the process. I was not complaining. I was suffering quietly.

A week later I went to see the oncologist. He saw me walking down the hallway.

"Theresa, what's wrong?" he asked.

"My legs are hurting me badly." The doctor realized that I did not need the booster shot because I am still young. The marrow in my bones produced at a good rate. The chemotherapy medication wouldn't necessarily affect my bones; being forty-eight years young worked in my favor.

The doctor gave me pain medication and some other medication for the nausea. The pain medication, Percocet, did help me, but the only thing that helped with the nausea was ginger ale and lime and my skittles; which I still eat. By the third week after treatment, my hair began to fall out.

What an experience. I will never forget it.

I was in the bathroom combing and styling my hair when I noticed that every time I ran the comb through my hair, there was hair left in the comb. I kept combing my hair and pulling the hair out of the comb and throwing it in the garbage. I did this repeatedly while staring in the mirror. I blanked out without realizing it.

My husband walked by the bathroom and saw what I was doing. I looked like I had zoned out!   He came in the bathroom and saw the amount of hair in the comb and in the garbage. He grabbed my hand, took the comb and pulled me out of the bathroom.

I just started crying. I melted in my husband's chest feeling so helpless because of what was happening to me. There was nothing that I could do about it. I had to learn how to deal with the enemy in the inner me.

I called my brother who is a barber. I explained what happened to my hair. He came over and cut the rest of my hair off. He was going to cut it in a short hair style, but he saw that as he cut my hair, it came off with very little help from his clippers. Literally, I could push my hair back and peel it off, just like you peel an orange. It was unreal!

Can you imagine that one day you have all this beautiful hair and the next day it's all gone? I was devastated. This was a traumatic experience. This disease affects the body in ways that are hard to describe.

I felt mortified through this whole process. It is a scary place to be in when you don't have any control of what you're going through and you really don't know what is going to happen next. It is very scary. I was always naked and up close and personal even when I didn't want to be. I would not have been able to go through this without the love, care and support of the best husband in the entire world. I know I mention my husband all the time, but I am extremely grateful for his love and his ability to stand by my side during a time like this.

I don't know how anyone could go through this alone. It's very challenging and difficult. I thank God for every cancer organization like The American Cancer Institute, and everyone who works to find a cure for cancer and other diseases.

I deteriorated right before my eyes and my family's eyes. It was debilitating. *Humiliating, too!* I could not believe that I was going through this! I did not know how to deal with the enemy taking over my body.

Have you ever gone through anything and asked yourself how am I going to get through this? I had a hard time accepting what life dealt me.

Did I do something along my journey that warranted this affliction?

I became afraid and angry. I knew within myself that my God was not punishing me with this disease. I knew God would get the glory out of my life. However, at the time, I did not see the blessing. I just saw the suffering.

I put on a good face. Oh yeah, I walked the walk, talked the talked, but I was so confused on the inside. I did not reason why I had to endure such pain. I could not digest what was happening to me. I felt like Data in Star Trek. "This does not compute."

I love God with all my heart and serve Him to the best of my ability. I just didn't get it!!

Can I be real with you?

There was really a war going on in my members – a war on the inside of me. The very thing I didn't want to think about, I thought about it. I thank God for knowing that the Lord is on my side even at times when I don't understand.

By the following treatment, I was completely bald. Every hair on my body was gone. The hair on my head, under my arms, my eyelashes, eyebrows, and my pubic hair were all gone in less than three weeks; what a scientific phenomenon.

Your hair is what defines you and gives you character. I didn't have long hair, but I had thick hair. My eyebrows were very thick and shapely; now all that was gone within three weeks of the first treatment.

I began to think about those who lived with the same enemy, the same disease that took over my body. Some people had support systems and others didn't. This is a disease that transforms your life without asking your permission. I couldn't believe that this was just the beginning of this enemy taking me over – physically, mentally and emotionally.

Oh my! There couldn't be more. Could there be?

I continuously thank God for my family. My brother, Dupree, the barber and his family as well as my brother, Prince who has his own mirror and glass business came over to support me during this time. At first, I was embarrassed. I did not want them to see me this way. They made me feel great even though I felt horrible on the inside.

I didn't like the way I looked or felt. They mentioned how cute I looked with a bald head. I was cute, but I didn't like being without hair. I thank God for being naturally pretty inside and out!

"Wow, your skin is as smooth as a baby's behind," my husband said.

He was right. It was as if I never had hair at all. I felt so awful inside. The support and love of my family encouraged me. It was the only way I was able to handle my new look and not be ashamed.

That evening we all spent time together laughing and enjoying our family. We were not hindered by time. We enjoyed each other's presence. I was glad to be alive and in their presence.

Family is a wonderful word. It's a union of people. Don't let anybody tell you differently; family is very important. It's God's foundation. The foundation of a strong family and God's unchanging hand has brought many generations through turbulent times. And when you don't have a blood relative, God places someone in your life that you are able to call family.

I love my family and I thank God for their support and most of all for their love for me. The words of a song come to mind, "Love lifted me, love lifted me, when nothing else could help, love lifted me."

The evening came to a close. I didn't want it to end because it kept my mind off of my journey with the enemy. Everyone left and we got ready for bed. After being diagnosed with breast cancer, my nights seemed so long and uncertain. I didn't know what God had in mind for me. God seemed very quiet. My mind and thoughts were working overtime.

~ ~ ~

By the third week, I almost felt like myself again. I was able to get up, make dinner, and walk around a little more. I didn't even lie down until the family came home from work and school. On the other hand, my mother was diagnosed with renal failure.

Renal failure? Dialysis? Breast Cancer?

In one family? Almost unbelievable.

I couldn't focus on my mother a whole lot. She had her battle and I had mine. Sometimes she wanted to go for dialysis and sometimes she didn't. We were both handling our enemies the best way we could.

One of the best ways I learned to handle any situation is to pray. Even though I was not at my original home church, my present church family was very good to me and my family.

What I enjoyed the most was Sunday morning prayer. I love to pray. When I became a born-again believer, I desired to pray. I used to hear Bishop Eric Figueroa, Sr., Evangelist Cynthia McInnis before she became a First Lady, and Evangelist Tammy Vaughn pray. I would tell God that I wanted to have a prayer life like them.

I would read the word of God and learn scriptures from the Bible. When you pray the scriptures from the Bible, your prayer is more effective. You are speaking God's language and not your own. God responds to His word.

2 Chronicles 7:14 states, "If my people, which are called by my name, shall humble themselves, and pray, and seek my face, and turn from their wicked ways; then will I hear from heaven, and will forgive their sin, and will heal their land."

In those days, every time the church doors were opened or service was going on, my family and I were right there. I would pray with all my heart; whether there was one person or one hundred people at church. I came to reach God, pray for others, and myself.

God would move all the time. Prayer does change things when you allow God to work in your life. During this time, I needed God more than life itself!

~ ~ ~

At week four, it was time for the second treatment. I was not looking forward to it at all. Once again, I went by myself because my family had to work. There was just something about walking this walk – taking each treatment as it came – with God. As you already know, by this time, I was bald. I began to wear African turbans.

I wasn't one to wear wigs or makeup except for lip gloss and eyeliner; my husband loves that natural look on me. He always tells me how pretty I am. I just love that man!

I pulled into the oncology parking lot as discretely as possible because I did not want to bring attention to myself. I didn't want my co-workers to see me. I was glad that I was on disability. I would not have been able to go through chemotherapy and work. There are some people who go to work and take chemotherapy. I pray that God blesses them all because it takes a lot to endure this kind of treatment.

I gave the parking attendant my car key and went inside the building. As I walked I prayed to prepare myself for the second treatment. I got off the elevator at the second floor, signed my name at the desk and then sat down and waited for them to call my name.

I was here again. The episode of the first treatment ran through my mind. I was not in a hurry to experience the needle or feel the sickness that words cannot explain.

"Theresa Hart." The nurse called my name.

It was time. As the nurse greeted me, I prayed silently that my veins would act right today. I really didn't want to get a port. I had only two more treatments to go.

Lord, let my veins work, please!

During this process I talked to my body a lot. I encouraged myself through God's word. The Lord was the only one who really knew what I was going through.

"This treatment is to help prevent the cancer from resurfacing in your body," the nurse explained. This wasn't the first time I was informed of this, but one treatment was surely enough to endure.

I praise God that the nurse was good and she got it on the first try. Once the treatment started, I put on my CD player and read my bible. I couldn't go to sleep because they gave me Benadryl and it kept me wide awake.

I didn't meet and greet during these treatments. I didn't want to be there. I was mad that I was there so the less communication with people, the better it was for me. I wanted to be in and out of that building. I was so private. I had no choice. Four hours later, the treatment was done and I left immediately.

I got out of that building so fast that it was as if I was never there. The parking attendants were all very, very nice, polite, and caring. They knew the kind of patients they were dealing with. I thank God for people who have a caring heart; they helped to make this journey more pleasant. I never felt like I was an obstacle or that all eyes were on me.

I left the hospital grounds and went shopping. I really wanted to stop by my job and see my co-workers, but I was too ashamed. I wasn't ready to "Show and Tell" yet. I reminded myself to do what I needed to do within the next two days because by the second night and third morning, the pain and sickness were indescribable.

I knew I would be sick as a dog. My husband had to put his cologne on outside or in his car; I was so sensitive to smells and tastes. I only went outside when I had to. Nobody really saw me during this time. I only went out when I had to go for treatments, to see my doctors, and go to church.

My husband is the best husband ever. He was right by my side through the toughest time in my life or should I say our lives. He was so caring; he made me laugh to take my mind off of what I was going through. He held me when I needed it; he gave me my space when I needed it, as well. The best part of this whole ordeal was that he was there.

Kevin was never selfish. He did everything in his power to make me comfortable. He made it all look so easy. I don't think too many people questioned him; they commended him and they were proud of him. If it was hard for him, the only one that knew that was God.

To have my husband stand by me during this sickness was priceless. A good support system is critical for a person's recovery. I have heard stories of families breaking up, people losing their minds, and people being selfish and not being able to handle the pressure of the sickness. They think about their own needs more than the one that is suffering with the disease.

When a person is sick for an extended period of time, it can become very challenging for family members. Truthfully, what happens is that their lives get put on hold and the person who is sick becomes the center of attention. Like it or not. It's all about the one going through the cancer or whatever trial life has dealt them.

Whatever the sickness or enemy, it's not good for a person to be alone through any difficult situation. We may play it off as if we don't need anyone. *Yeah, right!* We all need somebody to lean on and someone to understand us. Thankfully, I have it all; a wonderful husband, beautiful children, a loving church family, awesome co-workers, neighbors, and the best of friends.

Three days after the second treatment, I was so sick that I couldn't get out of bed. I hated to get up to go to the bathroom across the hall, but I did it anyway. I washed up, made my bed, dressed myself, ate a little and then lay back down in the bed. I forced myself to do these things. At this time, I was unable to physically help my mother, who was going through renal failure and dialysis. Needless to say, I put up a lot of prayers to God to heal both of us.

The best part of the day was when my family came home. My son came in from school and gave me the best hug. That hug was therapy for me. There wasn't a day that went by that I didn't receive my hug from my wonderful son. Before he did anything, I was his first priority. I love you, Bigboy!

I thank God for allowing me to also have a daughter because we can share almost everything. Even when I didn't say anything she already knew what I wanted and how I wanted it. When she came home from work, she came into my room to check on me. It hurt her like crazy to see me like that, so her way of dealing with it was to stay busy. She made sure the house was right. I trained her so well I didn't have to worry about keeping things in order. Nikki helped me with woman stuff. She bought clothes and items that she knew I liked. I didn't have the energy to go shopping anymore.

Nikki always checked on me. She looked in on me when I slept, bathed and at my doctor's appointments. Whatever I couldn't do for my mother, she was there to stand in the gap. She wasn't selfish. She helped her father with her brother and she went shopping and washed the clothes; she did it all. Thank you, "First born". I love you to life.

When my husband came home, he came in the room and gave me a kiss as he did and still does every day. I have known my husband for thirty-two years and there hasn't been a day that he hasn't called me or I have called him around lunch time. A lot of my co-workers could vouch for that. They used to say, "Theresa, Barry White is on the phone."

We prayed together every morning before he left to go to work. Then he made sure that I had everything I needed. I was thankful he was home, and that he loves me the way he does, and how our love continues to grow.

By the third treatment I was drained. I was weak. I looked like the life was going out of me. People were so kind and loving, but I know how I looked. The glow, the brightness, and the energy were no longer there. I was so, so, very tired. My oncologist told me to rest when I was tired. My stomach was so unsettled that everything made me sick. I lost weight rapidly. Ginger ale and skittles were my favorite food items.

I had to make myself eat. I drank a case of water in a week. In my mind I was trying to wash the chemotherapy medication out of my system. My mouth tasted like I had metal in it all the time. I moved around real slow. My husband and my daughter took me to my appointment because I could not drive. I was unable to push myself to do things. The doctors encouraged me not to push myself. My body was already fighting and I didn't need the stress or anything added to what I was dealing with.

If my body could talk, it would probably have told me off. *"Why are you torturing me, Theresa?"*

My body could not process the drastic change it went through. My body felt confused and so did I. I kept asking God, "What is this and why am I going through this?" I would just burst into tears. I didn't want anybody to see me like that. I didn't even have the energy to listen to my CDs or read the bible. I would just sit and pray and look at the TV. I really didn't know what was playing on the TV; it was just something to look at.

Finally, the day of the fourth and final treatment came. I was there.

Hallelujah. Glory to God! I made it alive?

WOW. I was so full of joy that I didn't even feel the pain. The feeling I felt when I walked through those doors was relief. I thought, *This is the last time I will walk through these doors!* The gift of life is more precious than the most valuable possession. You can't replace it and you can't get it back once it's gone. Therefore, choose to live and not die. Take this life that God has given you and show His glory through your life. What better way to be remembered than to make your life count by helping someone else's life matter. We all matter to God.

For the first time I didn't care how I was going to feel after the treatment; I knew this was it. Although, it was four treatments, it was really sixteen weeks of chemotherapy because the medication was so strong they had to give it to me in four cycles, three weeks apart. If not, I think the medication alone would have been too much for my body to handle at one time. I was extremely glad that it was over!

CHAPTER FIFTEEN
Radiation Therapy

After receiving four cycles or sixteen weeks of Cytoxan and Taxotere, it was now time to prepare for radiation. In the Radiation department, I underwent a CT-guided simulation to the area of the left breast. I went through an Intensity-modulated radiation therapy (IMRT) planning technique utilized to minimize the exposure to the lung and heart in the radiation field.

According to NYOH (New York Oncology & Haematology), CT Simulation utilizes computerized imaging technology that pinpoints the exact area to be treated. Three-dimensional pictures of the target-area are created and treatments are planned that precisely shape the radiation beam. This allows for individualized treatment plans to be developed that specifically target the tumor while minimizing the effect on normal tissue.

In other words, I had to have four pin-drop tattoos around the left and right sides, underneath my breast, and in my left armpit. I felt like a pincushion. For nearly two months, I received radiation therapy to the left breast. To be honest with you, it was so humiliating every time I went for a radiation treatment. I changed into a gown, and then I had to take it off to slide into my personally made cast. They positioned me in a way that the radiation would zoom right into the area where I had the cancer.

I tolerated this treatment well, in general, but it was a humbling experience. I had no privacy. My life was now an open book. I felt naked and exposed. I had thirty-six treatments, Monday through Friday. Everybody knew me, the doctors, the technicians, the nurses, and the patients like myself.

The stories I would hear were so overwhelming. I remember one story of a patient who received radiation therapy in her mouth because she had cancer in her mouth. As she came for therapy, her daughter would say how hard it was to get her to come because as the treatment continued, it got worse and it was hard for her to eat, drink, swallow and taste.

When you receive radiation treatment, the radiation builds up in your system, mainly in the area that's being targeted. I could only imagine what this woman was going through. My left breast started to get bigger and bigger. Then it started to get darker and darker.

Great! All the hair on my body is gone because of the chemotherapy treatments. Now, I am going to look even worse - my left breast looks abnormal.

I really put my husband through the test. At first I went to bed covered up because I was so ashamed of how I looked. I didn't feel pretty anymore. I didn't feel attractive, either. It was very difficult trying to please and love my husband. I couldn't even stand to be touched. My skin felt like it was burning all the time. I was so sensitive. By the twentieth treatment, I was burnt.

With the radiation building up in my system, my large breast looked even bigger, like a big black balloon. It looked like it was going to burst at any moment.

This is what I have to go through to get better...really?

I was burnt so badly that they had to put burn patches on me. My wonderful husband saw how I was suffering inside and out. Kevin has seen me at my best and my worst and yet he loves me even the more. He told me that he prayed to God to help him deal with this and to be able to go through this with me.

My breast was so sensitive that I could hardly stand for anything to touch the skin. So one day my husband, in his wisdom, took an old blue shirt and cut two holes in it where the breasts would fit. I put the shirt on, put my breasts through the holes, looked in the mirror and started laughing hysterically. My husband laughed, too. I called my daughter in the room to see what her father had created for me.

When she saw me in my newly-created shirt, she laughed. We laughed with each other. I looked so funny. Really! I had a bald head, now a t-shirt with holes in it for the breasts. I was something to look at. You know, I didn't take it as an insult in any kind of way. I know he did it out of the kindness of his heart. He was looking for a way to make his wife as comfortable as possible. It wasn't about the look; it was about being comfy and Kevin, made it happen for me every time. What God has given me in a husband like him is priceless.

This has really been a mind-changing experience. The way I see life now, I live each day as if it's my last. I love everyone, help anyone, and pray for everybody.

One day I went for the radiation treatment; I don't know what came over me. I got so emotional that I couldn't stop crying. I just felt tired, sore, and overwhelmed. By then, I'd had thirty-one treatments. I only had a couple of days left. Praise the Lord. I was almost at the finish line.

The doctor so understood my emotional pain.

"It's okay; you've been through a lot, Theresa. It's better out than in," she said. She took as much time with me as I needed. She wasn't in a rush to see the next patient; I had her undivided attention. All jokes aside, I was really hurting and there was nothing I could do about it other than to just go through it and not give up. The will to do will make a way.

"Are you still working?" the doctor asked.

"Yes, and it's very hard to move around," I answered.

"Oh no, Theresa, you shouldn't be working like this. I am writing a note for you to be out for a week. You need to rest and let your body heal after radiation. After the radiation it will take about five days before you will start feeling like yourself."

I was grateful to the doctor. I tried to be strong during the last couple of weeks because my husband was going through so much on his job. I didn't want to put any more pressure on him. I just wanted this to be over. My body was tired of hurting. The only time I had any relief was when I took pain medicine and before I went to bed, when I took a sleeping pill to help me sleep and be comfortable. Other than that, I was in so much pain.

Lord, how much of this can I take?

Part of me was a little selfish. I wanted all the attention and time, but I had to share it with the ones I love as well. I had to share in other life situations in my household and other things that were going on with other people in my family. Sometimes when you are sick, it's hard to put your attention on anything else other than what you are dealing with. At that point in my life, I needed constant help and encouragement. I knew my family was there for me, but I also felt so alone.

CHAPTER SIXTEEN
Marriage, Sexuality and Cancer

I have been married almost thirty-three years. We have had some tough days, some perplexing situations, but nothing prepared us or matched the travail that this disease, cancer, caused.

Truly our love for each other was on trial and our faith was pushed beyond our own intellectual capacity. It was the love of God and the love that we have for each other that prevented tragedy. This is not the kind of love that the world calls love, but, rather love that is pure, innocent, caring, uplifting, unselfish, daring to be different, daring to uphold a standard, compassionate, and letting nothing stand in the way of what is right according to the word of God.

Ephesians 5:22-33 (KJV) states,

> 22 Wives, submit yourselves unto your own husbands, as unto the Lord.

23 For the husband is the head of the wife, even as Christ is the head of the church: and he is the saviour of the body.

24 Therefore as the church is subject unto Christ, so let the wives be to their own husbands in every thing.

25 Husbands, love your wives, even as Christ also loved the church, and gave himself for it;

26 That he might sanctify and cleanse it with the washing of water by the word,

27 That he might present it to himself a glorious church, not having spot, or wrinkle, or any such thing; but that it should be holy and without blemish.

28 So ought men to love their wives as their own bodies. He that loveth his wife loveth himself.

29 For no man ever yet hated his own flesh; but nourisheth and cherisheth it, even as the Lord the church:

30 For we are members of his body, of his flesh, and of his bones.

31 For this cause shall a man leave his father and mother, and shall be joined unto his wife, and they two shall be one flesh.

32 This is a great mystery: but I speak concerning Christ and the church.

33 Nevertheless let every one of you in particular so love his wife even as himself; and the wife see that she reverence her husband.

This is God's prescription for marriage; anything less than this and you are missing out on His divine revelation in sharing your life with what God put together. God has given Kevin and me just that. God has shaped our love and relationship in such a way that we are a model family to be patterned after.

My husband is a gift from God to me. Often I ask myself if it's possible for someone to love you so much it's almost too good to be true. Then I answer myself and say, "Yes, because I feel the same way about him."

During the time I was going through with the cancer, we did not have any sexual relations. At one point, I thought that part of my life was over. It made me and Kevin question if we would have to love each other another way. Wow, this was incomprehensible. This was what this enemy called cancer did to my body for a moment.

I tried to understand what was happening with my body.

Oh my God, this is taking away my womanhood.

This could not be happening.

I spoke to my doctors, to the psychiatrist, and others who understood this process. Everyone said that it was a temporary inconvenience, but my desires would come back.

What? Are you serious?

I never thought that your natural body chemistry could leave you like that. I didn't know that cancer, chemotherapy, and radiation could invade your body so much so that it could take away the very essence of pleasure. The love that we have for each other I knew it was love.

"We are going to pray. I'm going to pray and ask God to help me through this," Kevin said. "I asked God to take the desire and place it where it was needed the most."

That is truly true love. I couldn't even think about how he felt, even though I cared and wanted him just as badly as he wanted me, but at that moment the desire was gone. I missed the passion between us.

God taught us how to make love to each other in other ways. We always loved being with each other. However, we liked each other even more. We never get tired of each other. How wonderful is that! Making love and reaching ecstasy is for a moment, but being together and sharing life and experiences is for a lifetime. We had passion in a new way.

He made love to me every morning when he woke up and we prayed together and when he kissed me before he left to go to work. He made love to me when he prepared my food the night before and the only thing I had to do was to get it out of the refrigerator and warm it up in the microwave. He made love to me when he called me every day at lunch time to see how I was doing. He made love to me when he washed and ironed my clothes. He made love to me when he was only able to hold me in his arms. He made love to me every day, showing me more and more how much he loves me.

He made love to me by showing me love, patience and kindness every day. He was going through, I know he was—he had to be—because the one he loved was suffering and the only thing he could do was make me as comfortable as he could. And Kevin did just that. He held nothing back. He made love to me by washing, dressing, and preparing me just as if I did it myself.

He made love to me, not just my body, but me, Theresa. He saw me in my worst as well as my best times and never stopped loving me. He made love to me every day. I love this man to life because of all that he did and still does for me. I thank him all the time for going the extra mile. It feels so wonderful when someone loves you so much it makes you blush all the time. It almost seems unreal, but it's for real.

Of course there is a medical side to what Kevin and I had to endure. The American Cancer Society explains it well in *Sexuality for Woman with Cancer.*

> **Lack of desire:** Both men and women often lose interest in sex during cancer treatment, at least for a time. At first, concern for survival is so great that sex is far down on your list of needs. This is quite normal. Few people are interested in sex when they feel their lives are being threatened. When people are in treatment, loss of desire may result from worry, depression, nausea, pain, or fatigue. Cancer treatments that disturb the normal hormone balance can also lessen sexual desire. If there is a conflict in the relationship, one partner or both might lose interest in sex. Any emotion or thought that keeps a woman from feeling excited can interfere with desire for sex. Distracting thoughts can keep her from getting aroused. Her vagina then stays tight and dry, which can make intercourse painful.
>
> **Pain:** Pain is a common problem for women during intercourse. It is often related to changes in the vagina's size or moistness. These changes can happen after pelvic surgery, radiation therapy, menopause, or treatment that has affected a woman's hormones.
>
> Sometimes the pain sets off a problem called vaginismus. If a woman has vaginismus, the muscles around the opening of the vagina become tense without the woman being aware of it. Her partner cannot enter the vagina. Pushing harder increases the woman's pain because her vaginal muscles are

> clenched in a spasm. Vaginismus can be treated with counseling and some special relaxation training.

When I read this the only thing I could do was cry. A sigh of relief came over me. It gave definition to the symptoms that I was going through. There were times that I did not know how to explain to my husband how I felt. I really thought it was all in my mind. Then I saw this book when I went for my three-month checkup with the oncologist. When I finished with the oncologist, I went to the second floor where I had chemotherapy to get a copy of my records; there was this book calling out to me to pick it up because the answers I was looking for were inside. I read it and realized that I was not losing my mind. These were the side effects my body had to go through.

Wow! I felt like I was a virgin all over again. I had to learn how to make love another way.

CHAPTER SEVENTEEN
Back to Work

There was one day I will never forget. I thought I was losing my mind. I didn't know what was going on inside of me. I was sitting at my desk at work and all of a sudden anxiety overtook me. I didn't know if it was the chemo, radiation, or the menopause; I needed to talk with someone right away. I thank God that I worked in the Psychiatry Dept. I asked to speak to one of the psychiatrists that I know. She didn't hesitate to speak with me. She knew what I had been through. I felt comfortable talking with her.

"Theresa, what's going on?" she asked.

"I don't even know. I feel so emotional, like I don't have control of myself. Everybody thinks that I'm this strong person, but I'm not!" I just began to let it all out. "I feel like my family and the people who know me think that because I finished the chemo and I appear to be doing well with the radiation that I'm okay. That's on the outside only, on the inside I am an emotional roller coaster. They really don't understand.

My husband has been there one-hundred-ten percent for me and even then he still doesn't understand. I am still trying to understand this myself. Sometimes he says he does; I tell him, 'Don't say that because you don't understand.' My children have been there for me; my son gives me so many hugs I can't count them and I need every one of them. My whole family has been there for me. I guess, I am doing better physically, but my emotions are spinning out of control." It all gushed out. I couldn't stop it.

She stated, "Theresa you have to realize you've been through a lot."

I shook my head. "I know. Sometimes I don't think about how much I've really been through. Even through all of this I have been able to maintain my responsibilities." I also told her that at the same time I was diagnosed with breast cancer; my mother was diagnosed with kidney failure. I told my family I could not handle taking care of my mother's illness and mine, too. No matter what support my brothers gave, my husband and I had to deal with a lot of my mother's care because she lived with us.

It was very hard. I guess I make everything look so easy, but it's not. Right then, I needed some definition as to what was going on inside of me. I am a person of control and I felt out of control.

"Let me do the scale with you," she said. "How is your mood?"

"Sometimes I am moody. Sometime I want to be bothered, but most times I don't." I continued to explain to her that even though I am a people person, I am a private person, as well. I like more one-on-one versus a group setting.

"Do you feel irritable?"

"Yes, my body is still going through a metamorphosis. My hands are numb, the heels on my feet are numb, and I have pain from my waist all the way down my legs."

She called it Neuropathy.

She continued asking questions, "How is your appetite?"

"It's unpredictable. I don't have my taste buds back from the chemotherapy yet."

"And how about sleeping habits? How do you sleep?"

"I rarely sleep. I am so uncomfortable." I started to cry.

"How's your motivation?"

"It's good. I like staying busy. It's therapy to me. Even though I need help, keeping up with my responsibilities takes my mind off of what I am dealing with."

As the psychiatrist continued to ask me various questions, I began to feel like I was not crazy after all. I just needed someone to help me sort things out. She helped me to talk it out and get it out of me so that I could characterize and prioritize my thoughts and feelings. When I left her office I felt better. I got a hold of myself again. Every now and then, I still go through this.

After being out for a week, I returned to work. I had my last radiation treatment (hallelujah), but the damage was already done. I had very bad rug burns on the left side of my breast where I had the surgery. I needed that week the doctor gave me to give my body rest and to let it heal naturally with the air hitting my breast, so I could get a skin on it.

On the day I returned to work, I had to go to employee health to be cleared to return to work. What an ordeal that was. My radiologist wrote a letter stating that I could return after a certain date; however, they needed a specific date on the letter. My appointment for employee health was at 7:30am and I was ten minutes early. I was the second one called, only to be informed that it wasn't going to be as smooth as I thought it would be. I had to leave and go to Radiation to get another letter. They were very nice at Radiation. They typed the letter and the doctor signed it right away. I fought with my emotions. It didn't take much for me to fly off the handle. If these people knew half of what I'd been through, all of that would not have been necessary.

I handed in the letter to administration and went to work as if I really wanted to be there. I wasn't ready to go back to work or to be around people. I wasn't comfortable with myself, yet. But, ready or not here I come! Everybody was glad to see me. I received many 'Welcome back' greetings and hugs, which were very comforting and genuine. It feels great when people really appreciate you for you. Not just what you can do for them or what they expect out of you, just you.

Between emails and phone messages, I had my work cut out for me. My co-worker sent me a reminder about a movie she had seen several months ago and reminded me it was playing that day. It was a film on breast cancer survival. The name of the movie is "Yona's Body". I replied to her message, but I was not sure if I was ready to look at this movie because my emotions and feelings were so unpredictable. I didn't feel like being vulnerable with myself.

The movie was at one o'clock in the Sloman Auditorium on the campus of the Zucker Hillside Hospital where I work. This film was part of National Women's Health Week. The movie was great! It was a wonderful illustration of what chemo and radiation do to the inside as well as the outside of the body. For some who have never gone through it, nor have had firsthand experience with someone being diagnosed with breast cancer, it is truly an awareness tool for intervention. For others like me, who have been through it and are still going through the after effects of therapy, I was able to identify with it and even add to the woman in the film's story.

I felt my emotions rising when she started talking about her hair falling out and looking and feeling horrible. When they showed the animated effect of the chemo going in the vein, it was as if I felt it going in my own veins all over again. It's a cool and hot feeling that goes through your veins. Once it gets into your system, which takes about two days to do so, your body begins to yell at you saying,

"What in the world are you doing to me? What did you put in me? I don't understand what kind of medicine this is. What kind of therapy is this? Help! I can't take all of this!"

Your body goes through withdrawal and an actual breakdown. The movie showed all of this in an equally funny and serious way. I pray as you read this book that you will have a better understanding and insight into this challenging disease.

~ ~ ~

I came to work with my blue turban on and before 10am I had pulled it off my head. The temperature was 90 degrees, but under my turban it felt like 110 degrees. Between the heat outside and the heat inside, I just took my turban off right at my desk and said, "It is what it is!"

I told myself, "Everybody is going to have to get used to me without my turban; I'M NOT WEARING IT ANYMORE!"

When my co-workers saw me, they all said I looked beautiful.

"You have the head and face to wear your hair short."

"You look so sexy, I wish I could wear my hair like that."

They didn't know what happened when they complimented me. It gave me more confidence and the boldness to be me.

I remember when I couldn't wait for five o'clock to come. I would take off the turban in the car. If it was cold I couldn't wait to get in my house and take the turban off my head. Those days are over, hallelujah!

It was a little funny to watch those who've only seen me in my turban. Their facial expressions told the story "That's how she looks without the turban?" or it could have meant "She looks very nice without her turban." They would just say 'Hi' or 'Good

Morning' looking at me, but not looking at me. I said to myself, "This too shall pass."

I felt a little uncomfortable that my hair was salt and pepper at forty-nine years old. I could not color or put any chemicals in my hair yet. I had to wait nearly three months. I didn't look or feel old, but everybody made me feel so good.

One person said, "Girl you have more pepper than salt." It felt great unwrapping. I sound like I'm speaking of a piece of candy. It is incredible the stages you go through as you get back to being yourself. I realized something; I will never be the same again. This is the new and improved Theresa!

~ ~ ~

I began attending a support group, but due to the holiday it was closed on this particular day. I missed the group, but I took the opportunity to go for a walk. I went to Home Depot and bought some carpet freshener and wax for the wood floors. It felt wonderful to get out and walk. I took my time getting to the store. I planned and made a blueprint in my mind of the things that I would do for myself and my family. It really felt good getting around on my own.

Often, we don't even appreciate the simple things in life. Walking, talking, getting around on your own and enjoying life. When I made it back home, I put the carpet freshener down and let it seep into the carpet. Then my husband vacuumed the rugs for me because that would have taken all of my energy. I waxed the floor. I just had to do the living room and the hallway. It came out beautifully, if I do say so myself! It felt good doing things I would normally do on a regular basis. Since being diagnosed with breast cancer, I've had to take one thing and one day at a time, because I get tired so fast. Nevertheless, I continue to tell myself that, "This too shall pass and my health is improving; better yet, this is the new and improved Theresa Hart!"

~ ~ ~

After all my treatments were done and the healing process began, it was time for a follow-up visit with the oncologist. I had a lot of questions. I needed to write them down. The side effects of going through breast cancer, taking chemotherapy and radiation, along with going through menopause have caused short term memory loss and chemo-brain. The following is what I wrote out to remind myself to ask the doctor during the visit:

- I am still feeling neuropathy in my fingers and legs.
- My vision seems different.
- I have aches and pain in my joints, knees, and shoulder.
- I am unbalanced.
- Everything seems more evident on my left side. I feel one sided at times.
- My appetite is off and on.
- I drink a lot of water.

- I get tired very easily - weakness and fatigue. How do I fight lingering fatigue? Taking a multivitamin? By eating more protein?
- Menopause is working overtime - night sweats, hot flashes, mood swings.
- Chemo-brain - I forget all the time. I have memory shortage and the inability to focus.
- One minute I am full of anxiety and sometimes feel out of control, then the next minute I channel that anxiety and do something positive, but it doesn't work all the time. Help…all of this is new.
- Stressful event – my mother doesn't do what she is supposed to do; I can't look after her and me too!
- What to eat to prevent the recurrence of cancer?
- Will I ever have a regular sex life again?
- When will I feel like me again?
- I need something for pain, sleep, and aching joints.

Unbelievable, I wrote it out, typed it, and still forgot it. When I got to the doctor's office I practically emptied my pocketbook in the examination room to find my notes. By the time the doctor's assistant came in the office I was so upset. I talked about how I couldn't remember the simple things anymore.

A woman like me, who previously could remember everything, couldn't remember from one minute to the next. I explained I just wanted to feel like myself again. I was tired of being in pain, tired of being uncomfortable, and tired of not being able to remember things. She assured me that it's normal and it's going to take time. She advised me not to rush it. "Look at it like this, the worst is over."

By that time the doctor came in the office. He was happy to see me, but when he looked at my face he said, "What's wrong, Theresa? When I saw you in the hallway the other day in passing, you looked wonderful and had a big smile on your face."

"I know. That day I was feeling great, but today I am not feeling so well." I explained to him the same thing I told his assistant. "I just want the pain to stop; I want to feel like Theresa again." He explained as well that I would get there little-by-little. He stated he want to do a CAT scan with contrast (a dye added through a vein or the rectum to see the targeted area better) of my brain and try a medication called Neurontin that would help with the nerve pain.

When I got home I called to schedule the CT scan with contrast of the brain. They wanted to know if I could come in on Saturday, but I said no because of the holiday weekend. I was looking forward to resting since we had to cancel the barbeque for the mentoring program that I run. Most of the children's families had plans or were going out of town for the holiday. We were not doing anything for the first time since we got the house. I just wasn't up to it.

I got an appointment for the CAT scan the following Monday. After the results came back, I received a call, "You have a beautiful brain." I still complained about being in pain. I just wanted my body to stop hurting! They prescribed the medication Neurontin. I took one at bedtime as prescribed and when I woke up the next morning, I felt horrible. I called the doctor from work and said that I was not taking it anymore because I did not like the way it made me feel.

"You have to get used to the medication."

"I do not want my body to get used to this medicine," I replied.

Had I not gone through enough?

~ ~ ~

Denise, my co-worker made a deposit in my life I was not expecting. She emailed me at work.

Denise: Hello. Are you there?

Me: Yes, I am here!

Denise: Ok, do you have a minute? If yes, I'm coming over for a minute.

Me: Yes!

Denise: Ok! I'm coming over.

I did not know why she wanted to come over all of a sudden. It wasn't the norm. I began to pray. To my surprise she had a gift for me. She told me that the Lord pressed upon her heart to do this. She took it out and gave the gift to me. It was a book with the title "The Enemy in the Inner Me". I said to myself, *Wait a minute this is the title of my book.* I looked at the book and the bottom read, "by

Theresa Hart". I was in shock. It was as if I was looking at my future; it was right in my face.

I was overwhelmed with thanksgiving and so grateful that someone thought about me. She did not want anything, but she poured into my life. What a blessing. I remember when Denise did this before. She gave me a silverware set with an invitation to my housewarming party. A house that was nowhere in sight, yet. Within a year of the gift God had blessed us with a house. I really have to be careful what I say out of my mouth around some folk!

A few weeks later my family went on vacation. On the third day of our trip, my husband, Kevin ruptured his Achilles tendon. He made it through the vacation on my medication until we returned home. Nikki took him straight to the emergency room when we came back. They put a brace on it and told him to see an orthopedic doctor. When Kevin met with him, the doctor told him that he had to have surgery. I could not believe what I was hearing.

Not Kevin! Surgery? Are you for real?

I was not healed yet!

~ ~ ~

A few months later, I woke up with a praise of thanksgiving to God on my lips and a new outlook on my life. It was a rainy day, but that didn't bother me at all. The night before, I began to read, *The Uncommon Leader: 31 Keys for Unlocking your Greatness* by Dr. Mike Murdock. I was encouraged by just the first few lines.

When I opened up the book the first thing I read was, "Winners are simply ex-losers who got mad." Praise the Lord! I needed to have read this a while ago. He also stated, "Circle today's date on your calendar and declare that the happiest and most productive day of my life is beginning today!" So I woke up with a renewed spirit in the Lord.

I had an appointment with the oncology doctor. I hadn't been to that office in over a year! Almost a year later…look at God! I bless His name for His awesome power, favor, grace, and mercy towards me. I thank God for healing my body of breast cancer. I will say this until I die!

I did not understand why this had to happen to me, but as I look back, I realize that to be able to tell the story of being a survivor is a testimony all by itself. As I sat there in the doctor's office waiting for them to call my name, I no longer felt mortified about how I looked.

I didn't feel like everyone was looking at me because I had the "cancer look". The last time I was here I had a turban on my head, my nails were black, and I was sick to my stomach. My body, mind, and soul were recovering from the shock of cancer as well as going through chemotherapy and radiation. My body was recovering from CAT scans, PET-scans (a radioactive test that looks for disease), MRIs, mammograms, sonograms, had my blood drawn every week and was taking all kinds of medications. My body needed a breather from everything.

Glory to God! The joy that I felt right then in my soul, words can't describe the thanksgiving I felt and the love I have for my Jesus. Receiving this blessing is like Heaven on earth. Money could not help, my family was limited in their support, my friends were limited in their support, but the grace of God rested on me and God knew what I needed even when *I* didn't know what I needed. He brought me through the hardest time of my life. I heard a Bishop say, "When you can't feel God's hand, know God's HEART, and when you can't feel His presence, know His Omnipresence!"

As I sat in the doctor's office waiting to be seen, I couldn't stop thinking about that statement. I have so many testimonies in my life and my families' lives that I know that the Lord loves me. So in a way I do know His heart; I know he would never leave me or forsake me. We will go through life's roads, hills, and valleys, but I thank God that He is with us every step of the way.

CHAPTER EIGHTEEN
The Turning Point

And Hannah prayed, and said, my heart rejoiceth, in the Lord, mine horn is exalted in the Lord, my mouth is enlarged over mine enemies; because I rejoice in thy salvation.
1 Samuel 2:1

I attended a Women's Conference at New Life Tabernacle – the church that I realized later on that I should not have left. The guest speaker, Evangelist Cynthia McInnis preached a message that lined me up with my destiny with God. The title of her message was, "Can You Hear Me Now?" taken from 1 Samuel 1:13-17

13 Now Hannah, she spake in her heart; only her lips moved, but her voice was not heard: therefore Eli thought she had been drunken.

14 And Eli said unto her, How long wilt thou be drunken? put away thy wine from thee.

> 15 And Hannah answered and said, No, my
> lord, I am a woman of a sorrowful spirit: I have drunk
> neither wine nor strong drink, but have poured out my
> soul before the LORD.
> 16 Count not thine handmaid for a daughter of
> Belial: for out of the abundance of my complaint and
> grief have I spoken hitherto.
> 17 Then Eli answered and said, Go in peace:
> and the God of Israel grant thee thy petition that thou
> hast asked of him.

When no one knows what's going on with you, they will always draw their own conclusion about you. That's why you don't always let your right hand know what your left hand is doing.

When she finished the message and ministered to me in my ears; some words were only meant for me to receive what God was saying through Evangelist McInnis. I knew I had to make a move, I just didn't know how to do it.

When you are upset you don't think, you can't react and don't really take into consideration all of the people you may affect. I needed God to lead me this time. This message was as if God was yelling from heaven "CAN YOU HEAR ME NOW?"

It was the turning point for me. I knew God was turning my situation around and touching the heart of all who were affected by me leaving my church – it was a wrong decision.

I was so overwhelmed. The next thing I knew, I was on the wall weeping and wailing, but when I got up, I got up with the victory and thanked God for another chance.

~ ~ ~

I received a call from the hospital around 12:30am letting me know my mother was having trouble breathing and they had to put her on a breathing machine. While the doctor talked, I got dressed. The doctor needed my consent to put a catheter in her groin area because they had trouble with her veins.

Going back and forth to the hospital and seeing my mother in this condition was difficult to walk out. She's my mother; you only get one, and regardless of the relationship, she's the one that brought you into this world.

For over two weeks, there was no change in my mother's condition. The doctor spoke to me about performing a tracheotomy because my mother couldn't stay on the ventilator for a long period of time.

When he said 'tracheotomy' my heart felt like it skipped a beat. As I listened to what he was saying, I thought to myself about how my mother had been through so much. As if dialysis was not enough, now she needed help breathing.

Lord, how much more will she be able to take?

My mom had the surgery. Even though my faith and trust were in God and He assured me that she would be okay, my emotions were all over the place as I waited to hear the results from the doctor.

On the same day, I had an appointment for my mammogram and sonogram after treatment with chemo and radiation. "Praise the Lord!" I gladly pronounced that "I have the VICTORY!" I received a good report that all was clear and there was no cancer in my breast. "Thank God!" I waited patiently to hear the same praise report for my mother.

In the midst of all of this, our family battled with our spiritual growth and where our hearts were in regards to where we would attend church. Just a word of wisdom; never make a move or any decision when you are hurt or angry.

~ ~ ~

I received a phone call from the hospital informing me that they'd had to intubate my mother because her trache was clogged with thick mucus and they could not suction her. When I received the news, I broke down at my desk on my job. She was doing so well a few days before. My sister-in-law had gone up to see her. She had done her hair and spent some quality time with her. I could not wait to get up to the hospital to see her that day.

When I walked in the room, I said, "Look at you, who did your hair?"

To my surprise my mother answered, "Leveda."

I was in shock to hear her speak. "And you're talking now, wow!"

I had told everyone how great she looked and that she had even had some water to drink. Afterwards I had called the doctor to inform him about my mother's progress and he'd changed the order of the feeding tube that was going to go in her stomach.

Now it seemed like we were right back where we started; but the "devil is a liar". It was a temporary inconvenience for a better improvement.

"Mommy, it's okay. You had a little setback, but this is only temporary." Her eyes welled up with tears and rolled down the side of her face. I cried as well.

As much as I tried to be strong for her, it was hard that day because none of us expected this. I explained to her that over the weekend, they would put the trache back in and put the feeding tube in her stomach to prepare her to leave the hospital and go to the rehabilitation center. She was glad to hear that.

She had the tracheotomy done that Saturday and they put the feeding tube in that Monday evening.

When my daughter and I went up to the hospital, we expected to see her sedated because she had just had a minor surgery done, plus she had dialysis the same morning. We thought she would be worn out, but she was bright-eyed and bushy-tailed.

We were surprised and excited at the same time to see that she was so alert. We stayed with Mommy until 10pm, talking, laughing, and making her feel excited to get out of the hospital. I knew she was looking forward to leaving more than any of us.

Soon after, my mother was admitted to a rehabilitation center.

~ ~ ~

As I prepared to close out the year, I looked forward to the new year with no limits or boundaries. This was a healthy beginning for me. It was an icy December day and I was the only one going to work. I had exhausted all of my time on disability for six months due to the breast cancer. I had to go back to work for financial reasons and to build up my time at work.

Still recovering in my body, mind, and spirit, I had to muster up strength to go to work. In my mind, I thought about church and how I was looking forward to going that night. I was stepping out of the old into the new. Praise the Lord.

When you go through a struggle, you are always looking for a way out to feel better. I went to the post office before I went to work, sent off a package for my brother and wished everybody a Happy and Healthy New Year. Why can't we greet one another like this every day? There's something about the new year; out with the old and in with the new. It was so bad outside I couldn't even make it to work. It was so icy that people were running into each other. Nobody had control on the ice. I turned the car around and came home. I called and let my job know I was not going to be able to make it in due to the weather. I made it back home safely. This gave me more time to prepare for the new year. The bible says, in Revelation 3:2, "Strengthen those things which remain."

I was looking forward to strengthening what remained. When you go through so much you don't think anything is left. Only God knows this inner struggle. I missed me, I really did. I used to be full of energy, able to multitask, and loved all of it. Now it's hard for me to complete one task, but He will strengthen that which remains. What I had is more than enough with God.

It was around 9:30pm on New Year's Eve and my family and I were on our way into a new beginning. I was so excited on the inside that I was ready to burst! Having a change and a new beginning meant so much to me that I can't explain it. I knew God had a plan for my life. I am alive, and God gave me another chance. I'm excited about what God will do in my life.

I'm here on purpose. Glory to God! God, I love you for all the blessings you have given to me. I made it to another year. Thank you, Jesus!

Although the year started out well, I still had some obstacles to face. I did not realize this healing process was going to be so long.

My faith was on trial, again.

When God? When will this pain go away?

I am tired of suffering in my body.

This pain is so tiresome.

I had to deal with mother's health and accept the fact that she was going to need long term care. I was so used to caring for her that now we had to care for her in a different way.

In the process of caring for my mother, my back started to fail me. I thought it was stress, but I soon found out that I had a bulging disc pressing against my spine.

Great! When will it end?

I began physical therapy and had to get injections in my back. When it rains it pours, so they say. For the last five months of the year, I went out on disability again.

I silently went into a depression. I was confined to my bedroom. The only time I came out was when I had to go to the doctor and when we went to church. I smiled on the outside and appeared to be functioning well in life, but I was not doing a good job.

Then the unimaginable happened; my daughter got sick.

~ ~ ~

My love was sick and she didn't even know it. She was losing weight, but for some reason her stomach wasn't getting flat. So without saying anything to me, she went to a women's clinic because at the time she didn't have medical insurance. She had recently opened her daycare business; none of us saw this sickness coming.

When she returned home, the look on her face was uncertain. The doctor that examined her said "What is this?" and "What are you into?"

My daughter replied, "What do you mean?" That was a strange comment from the doctor. The doctor said she had never felt what she felt inside my daughter, so she really didn't know what to say. My daughter explained how another doctor came in and stated she needed to have a sonogram and some other tests done.

When she came home and told me what was going on, I couldn't believe my daughter was going through something like this. She sat on the couch and told us everything. My family touched and agreed and laid hands on her stomach and proclaimed, "Devil, you are a liar!" and commanded him to, "Get your hands off my baby."

The Lord led me to tell my daughter to call my OB/GYN. I know it was meant to be because everything fell into place once she did. We soon found out that my daughter had a fibroid that needed to be removed from her uterus.

I thank God for my church family, New Life Tabernacle. My Bishop Figueroa, First Lady Doreen Figueroa, and the whole church family prayed the prayer of faith and healing for my daughter. The surgery was a success. After the surgery my daughter walked out as if nothing had happened.

We thought it was all over, but to our surprise it was just beginning. It seems that when the doctor took out the first fibroid, the other fibroid began to grow and grow. As a result, my daughter had to have major surgery.

The fibroid grew to eight pounds. I did not understand why God was allowing these illnesses to happen in my family. When it happens to you, it's easier for you to handle, but when it happens to your child, it takes it to another level; and it takes a Holy God to give you the strength you need to get through.

The stress began to mount up. I was out on disability, my daughter had to have major surgery and we had to deal with her new daycare business. This was a lot to deal with emotionally. I will always say this, "If it wasn't for the Lord on my side, I would have lost my mind".

When you go through one trial after another, sometimes your strength grows small; but for some reason, in my weakness my strength became bigger than my problem. I didn't even realize it until I looked back on what we had been through. While I was in it I felt numb. I kept moving so I wouldn't feel anything, but I had my faith in God.

I kept encouraging my daughter because she would look in my face to see if there was any fear. When she saw my faith and confidence, it caused her faith and confidence to build in trusting God. She kept working until it was time for her to have the surgery and our church family kept praying the prayer of faith and healing.

Even though you may go through trying times in this life, it is better to have God present in your situation than to go through this life without Him at all.

My mother-in-law and I were with my daughter the day of the surgery. When the doctor came out of the operating room and said, "This is going to be a bloody mess" my heart skipped a beat.

"I explained everything to your daughter," she said. "I will do everything I can to save her uterus, but if I can't, to save her life, I will take it." When she went back into the operating room, my mother-in-law and I prayed. We were crazy enough to believe God that He was going to bring my daughter out on top and that's just what He did!

"When I opened her up, the fibroid popped right out," the doctor explained. "It was sitting on top of her uterus. It was so heavy it looked like it was in her uterus due to the weight of it." To God be the glory! The doctor showed us the pictures of the fibroid. It was the shape of a round watermelon. It was perfectly round.

"It was not a hard surgery; and there was little to no blood because it popped right out. It was a miracle," the doctor said.

Once again, God showed Himself to be powerful and great in our lives. Thank you, Jesus, for my daughter's victory. You must know that miracles still happen, when you believe.

CHAPTER NINETEEN
A New Beginning

I arrived at church late one Sunday morning. I don't like to make a habit of coming late, especially since I recently returned to my birthing place. We came in quickly and sat in the third row from the back. I did not want to bring attention to myself, but my Bishop told the ushers to bring us to the front.

We were in the front enjoying Jesus and getting caught up in the praise and worship; with my eyes closed I praised God because my heart rejoiced that it felt good being back at New Life Tabernacle. Lifting up my hands in true worship and with tears rolling down my face, I thanked God for His grace and mercy and being able to feel the anointing of God.

As I worshipped, I did not realize it, but Bishop Eric R. Figueroa, Sr., my pastor, came down from the pulpit and walked over to me. The next thing I knew, he laid hands on me and said,

"Theresa Hart, the Lord said you are going to preach the word of God."

Oh, I can still feel that overwhelming feeling that flooded my heart with so much love. God called me. He called me to preach His word. All I could do was praise God. I cried tears of joy and thanksgiving. I was not looking for anything. I was grateful to be called a child of God and it was enough for me; anything else is truly humbling. To be used by God is the best blessing that anyone can ask for.

~~~

> I took the call to preach seriously. It was an honor to preach the word of God and I was determined to do my very best. I will never forget my initial sermon. The scripture was Luke 22:31:32,
>
> And the Lord said, Simon, Simon, behold, Satan hath desired to have you, that he may sift you as wheat:
>
> But I have prayed for thee, that thy faith fail not: and when thou art converted, strengthen thy brethren.

The title of my initial sermon was, "Still I Rise".

Recently, my girlfriend, Pam sent me an email regarding the first black male valedictorian in ten years from Booker T. Washington High School. At the graduation, he spoke about being shot at, his mother going through cancer, and his brother dying. Yet, he stood before the people as the first black male valedictorian in over ten years and with over a million dollars in scholarships for undergraduate and graduate colleges.
~~~

This made me think about my own testimony. In the verses above, Christ wanted Peter to become aware of the devil's design (v 31). The Lord said, Simon, Simon, [watch, study, examine, observe] what I say; Satan hath desired to have you, that he may sift you as wheat.

The devil wants you so bad that he can taste it! He wants control over your life, your family, your finances, your body, your mind, and your soul—he wants all of you!

I wondered why Jesus only mentioned Peter when he had twelve disciples. In my studies, I learned that from the start Peter seemed to have been the spokesman for the other disciples, the man who stood out from the group. Peter is always mentioned first, which seems to show he was Jesus' right hand man.

Peter was an ordinary fisherman in Galilee, leading an ordinary life, he was very normal like the rest of us. Often, he was quick at the mouth or with his actions, bad-tempered and he would get very angry, but overall he was capable of great loyalty and love.

Peter was the one who was not afraid to speak out. Peter was one of the first disciples Jesus called. Jesus said, "Come with me and I will make you fishers of men."

It was Peter who saw Jesus walk on water and asked him, "Lord, if it be thou, bid me come unto thee on the water." And Jesus said, "Come." Peter walked on the water until he took his eyes off of Jesus.

When you take your eyes off the Lord, that is when you start to sink and everything starts to consume you. However, when you keep your eyes stayed on Jesus, miracles happen.

When Jesus asked his disciples, "Whom do men say that I am?" it was Peter who said, "Thou art the Christ, the son of the living God." Jesus told Peter, "Flesh and blood hath not revealed this unto thee, but my Father which is in Heaven." Matthew 16:18, Jesus says, "That thou art Peter, and upon this rock I will build my church; and the gates of hell shall not prevail against it."

Peter was aware of Jesus' divinity and he blurted it out, demonstrating his faith and insight. The charge Jesus gave Peter was to help others as Christ helps us. "When thou art converted, strengthen thy brethren…" Luke 22:32. This means when you recover by the grace of God, and are brought to repentance, do what you can to help others recover. Encourage others to hope that they also shall find mercy.

Those that have fallen into sin must be converted from it; those that have turned aside must return; those that have left their first love must do their first work and return to the Lord.

As a new minister of the gospel of Jesus Christ, it is my privilege to share with everyone my testimony of faith and healing. God preserved me to share his love with you. Many of us are like Peter, we live ordinary lives and are imperfect in so many ways, but God desires to do extraordinary things with us. God helps us to rise out of every situation that we encounter.

If you're reading this book, I am in the next chapter of my life. Life up to this point has been a priceless lesson. As Oprah Winfrey stated, "Life is a Class". Life is the best gift that God has given us. What we do with it will determine how grateful we are.

I am ready to seize what God has in store for me. I want the whole world to know that you don't have to be defeated when you experience this type of sickness. There is a verse in the song, "So Happy Being Me" by Donald Lawrence that sums it up for me.

"Looking back on
When I started
Had a lot of sun
And a lot of rain,
I've had some joy
And been broken-hearted
But now that doesn't... mean a thing.
I'm living for the joy and laughter
I'm learning from my
Before's and after's
All in all, it's been cool
His grace, it brought me through
So happy being me, I'm regretting nothing
'Bout me
Too busy living life, giving love... freely
I'm so happy being me."

This has been "An Unexpected Journey" as my dear friend, Tina Gates put it. This breast cancer was designed to kill me, but God had another plan for my life. I'm reminded of a theme I wrote for the Boys' and Girls' Mentoring Program Chronicle newsletter. The title is "I Will Win!"

No matter what the trial, challenge, or test, I will win! Another year has ended and a new year is beginning. Oh, what expectation I have. I'm looking forward to. We have another chance to make a difference. We have a lot of areas to win in, put our best foot forward and work ten times as hard.

I will win! There were some challenging times; there were some close calls; our faith was tested by every sense of the word, yet, we made it! We made it! With God's grace and mercy, He's brought us into a new beginning.

Philippians 3:13 says, "Brethren, I do not count myself to have apprehended; but one thing I do, forgetting those things which are behind and reaching forward to those things which are ahead."

I always WIN!

CHAPTER TWENTY
Words of Encouragement

To my daughter,

I love you and am so very proud of you. You have always been a strong woman. Your brothers and so many others have looked up to you. Even though you have had some challenges and your plate has been full, you have been there for everybody. Now it's your time to shine. Let God bless you in a special way.

Love,

Your mother,

Lillie M. Pope

***

To my wife,

God bless you on this wonderful adventure. Letters or words of encouragement are developed in our minds every minute for those we love dearly. God has always had his hand of covering, favor, protection, on you since day one. You have mastered completion. Your body has been a centerpiece for God's healing powers. Continue to complete your journey. I will always be there!

Pure love,

Jack K. Hart "VC"

***

To My Wonderful Mother,

My mother does not play when it comes to her family and the need that is required to keep us together. My mother went to the doctor for a routine checkup only to find out she had cancer; notice I said had! Yes, God delivered her from this disease. I thank God that He has brought her out of this. My mother didn't know that it hurt me so bad to see her in pain and I couldn't do anything about it, but pray and comfort her with all the love I have for her.

My mother is a strong black woman. My mother has done some things she wasn't proud of, but her struggles helped mold her into the great woman she is today. When my mother had me she wasn't married, but trust and believe my dad and her made it right in the eyes of God. She has shown me through God that that is where her help and strength come from.

My mother is my role model. She shows me how to be a Godly woman and how to be a family woman. I don't see that in the world today. Family is just a word and marriage is a reality show. My mother and father have been happily married and in love with each other for 32 years. It's not just a picture; she lives what she talks about.

My mother is a woman of uniqueness. There is only one Theresa Hart. I love you so much my special lady of life. You are a wonderful mother, wife, friend, and mentor; whatever your hands find to do, you do it right well.

You are a prayer warrior and you rightly divide the word of God. You are a life giver and you show me what a Christian woman looks like. I love you, Mommy and I see the love that you put in everything that you do. You exposed this disease for what it really is; an enemy that God blessed you to defeat.

I can always count on you. You wear so many hats, that I pray when it's my turn, I make you proud.

This is to the wonderful lady of my heart. I love you, Mommy.

Your *daughter,*

Nikki, "First Born"

***

Hi Sister,

This is a letter of encouragement, for those who had or have a loved one with breast cancer. I am living proof that it hurts when a family member has cancer. My sister, Theresa had breast cancer. When you hear that word cancer, the first thing that comes to mind is that you are going to lose your loved one. However, as long as you believe in the Lord, praise God in it and let your loved ones know that you'll be on their side 100%, they will beat that cancer. I love my sister with all my heart. Losing you would have been like losing a mother.

Your brother,

Anthony Pope "Prince"

***

Theresa,

You are someone who prayed for their brothers because of the life we chose as teens. You are someone who started a free food program when people said it could not be done. When I found you were diagnosed with breast cancer, my life stopped for a moment and I said, "Out of all people, why her? One who prays for other people and has faith that God can fix all things. One who prays in her car before driving and she is someone who beat drug addiction." You hear about cancer on TV, the radio, and others going through cancer and you sympathize, but when it hits home it's hard to believe. We are talking about someone who prayed for her father that by the time he passed, he himself had a relationship with God and her brothers gave their lives to God. My sister went through this ordeal, yet God brought her through with His mighty hand. I know God will use this to bless other people's lives. God bless you, sis. Keep praying and allowing God to use you.

Love,

Dupree Pope, Baby Brother

***

Theresa,

May I take this inspiring moment to pause and say, "Congratulations!"

One of my memories during your illness was how you still maintained your dedication as a wife, mother, and a mentor to the family. How this has reached down and touched all of us. You can say with great assurance "I am in God's Favor".

Love,

Gladys Hart

Your Mother-in-law

***

Theresa,

As a teenager, you came into my life through a mutual friend, Reiko. I felt a sister bond from the first time we met. You were the sister I wanted.

I wanted it so bad I locked up your belongings when it was time for you to go back home. I was mad at you for leaving. I got over it and we have remained "sisters" through the years. I was diagnosed with breast cancer in 2006. I went through chemotherapy, radical unilateral mastectomy, and radiation. You were there the whole time encouraging and praying for and with me. On the day of my surgery, YOU are the one who brought me to Hackensack University Medical Center. You gave me the perseverance and energy to get through losing one of my magnificent "girls" with a positive outlook. I still have my prayer that your wrote for me. I read it often.

When you called and told me that you were diagnosed with breast cancer the bottom fell out. I felt awful, like it was my fault, like if you didn't take me for my surgery you would have been spared this dreaded disease. As usual, you told me I was being silly and that had nothing to do with it. You said the Devil is a liar and like me, you too will prevail. You were right! We have gone through trials and tribulations of a cancer diagnosis together. With the power of prayer and love, we have both made it through the dark days of chemotherapy, bald heads and nausea. Praise God!!

Marguerite Scott

***

Theresa,

I am a twenty-eight-year-old cancer survivor. I am a statistic that has beaten the odds. There are thousands of us each year. Each day we quietly celebrate life, we embrace each day with a thankful attitude and a blessed feeling. We have been face to face with our mortality. Survival skills vary, we do not have to travel the same route to get to the same destination but the important thing is that you, too, can survive. With medical support, prayer, spirituality, family and friends support, and most of all your steadfast faith in God, you, too, can be a survivor.

Delilah Green

***

Theresa,

When I think of this Scripture I always think of you: 2 Timothy 3:10-11 "But you have carefully followed my doctrine, manner of life, purpose, faith, longsuffering, love, perseverance, persecutions , afflictions, which happened to me...what persecutions I endured. And out of them all the Lord delivered me". It takes a strong, courageous, patient, and submitted woman of God to go through all that you've gone through without giving up. Even though I don't know all the things God has brought you through, I have some knowledge you endured is the kind of stuff that has created the brokenness, sharpens iron with iron, to bring forth by God's grace Pastors, true Evangelists, Ministers, and submitted leaders that God places strategically among us. This is one thing I do know that you deserve everything good that God has for you. It goes without saying that I am expecting even greater things for you and from you. Thank you so much, Theresa! I've been remembering how much you tried to encourage me by always telling me that I was more than making Sunday programs. I am very grateful to you for trying to stir the gift by putting me on your programs as a speaker. Theresa, I appreciate everything you have done for me-and now I guess I'll have to follow your example and allow myself to be broken so that I can serve God. Submitting to His purpose and plan for my life. You, Theresa, are a "hard act" to follow! I've always run from the "brokenness" but because of your testimony I see that the brokenness takes us to Victory and another level in Christ. Congratulations! Love you! Your daughter in Christ

Theresa Williams

***

Theresa,

"Experience is not what happens to you; it is what you do with what happens to you." I've watched you overcome many struggles with dignity and grace. Your story can and will encourage others to overcome their barriers to treatment. You've inspired me in many areas of my life. God Bless you and thank you for being my lifelong friend. Congratulations,

Diane

***

Theresa Hart put her interest to the test in creating a mentoring program for young boys and girls in the neighborhood of South Floral Park and Elmont in Long Island. She started out with few resources, and many facets were developed by trial and little errors. She recognized the benefit of using parenting skills as a part of her program. The responses of the children grew as they were included in planning projects to benefit the community and as they learned social and educational skills. When Theresa was diagnosed with breast cancer, it never stopped her love and responsibilities for the children. She is needed and her story is worth hearing.

Ms. J. Bradley

***

To Theresa Hart,

Continue to inspire all that you touch and meet with God's word and the experience and wisdom He has taught you. Stay on the path of your words of wisdom and continue on the path He has put you on. To God be the Glory!

Ms. B. R. Peterson

***

To Theresa aka Momma T,

I'm extremely proud of you and this new venture. You are a remarkable woman who I am very thankful to know. You have been a second mother to me and I can never repay or thank you enough for everything you've done for me; from advice to prayers. I know that this next chapter as an author will bring you continued blessing upon blessing. You are the epitome of a strong black woman; a wonderful wife, mother and friend. I love you and can't wait to see what else God has in store for your life!

Love,

Tiffany Taylor

***

Mother T,

Experience is not what happens to you; it is what you do with what happens to you. ~ Aldous Huxley

Your existence, your love, your support, your determination, and your spirit are passed on to all you have come in contact with. Thank you for being a proven link to what all can be done if you accept and believe. You are what I want to become; a better woman, mother, wife, sister, friend and community leader. Keep showing me the way. Keep uplifting me. You are the most beautiful spirit I will ever know. With love always.

Your inherited daughter,

Noelle D. Coote-Anderson

***

Dear Theresa,

I am writing to encourage you to hold steadfast and keep praying during this trying period. This is not an easy struggle for you, and I want you to know that I am all the way praying for your quick recovery. Your pain was not an easy one to bear, but God said, "If you only believe that I have the power to heal you, it will be done." Because you are a child of God, and He knows your innermost thoughts, He is able to help you to not think about the pain, but to say, "God, I trust You for who You are."

While you were in this struggle, and indeed it was a struggle, taking chemotherapy and radiation, I prayed for you. Sometimes while praying, tears flowed down my cheeks because I have experienced persons who have gone through chemotherapy and radiation. God spoke to you and said, "No more, my child. I am going to heal you quicker than you expect to be healed." This is a testimony for others that if you put God first, He will do the rest.

I will always love you,

Maggie Pollydore

***

Dear Theresa,

It is with great honor that I write this dedication for your book. I was so surprised with deep sadness to hear that you had cancer. I knew that your faith would see you through this trial. You walked the test of fire and came through without a mark. With this in mind I made a pink scarf as a symbol of your survival.

May God continue to bless you,

Pat

***

Theresa,

My co-worker, my friend, my sister, and my mentor to name a few, you truly are a child of God. You lift me up many days. I remember when you got ill how worried and troubled I felt. We would talk for periods of time on the telephone. You had such faith and conviction to win the battle with that disease. I was so happy when you returned to work. I decided we both were going to fight that demon by walking to get stronger and healthier. The first day up the road was very short. You went about a block and told me to go ahead and you would wait until I came back. Before I knew it, your distance progressed rapidly and we were walking side by side up the hill (smile). That was a good feeling. I remember one morning your daughter took you to work and you saw me walking, you got out of the car and joined me. Your humble child waited for us at the job.

I am forever grateful for your company,

Pauline Walker

***

My Dearest Friend Theresa,

It seems like a lifetime ago that you were diagnosed with breast cancer. When I heard it, it was such a shock! It was just the other day that you were laughing, baking your famous cheesecakes and selling those adorable flip flops. Yes, it seems like a lifetime ago that you had that most dreaded disease. I missed seeing you at work and the aroma of your perfume lingering in the hallways. It appeared as though you were never returning to work. Then one day you came in for a visit. Oh man! We all were so happy to see you, Theresa. Now I know you had to go through something that is so indescribable, but you would never know it with your Spirit! Even with your hair loss, at first you wore a wig every now and then, but when you got too HOT and off that went! To me you looked beautiful with your short hair. Before we knew it you were back to work; maybe not a full day but it was a start. Then you were really back, laughing again, cooking your cheesecakes and being the beautiful person that you are. I thank GOD for you, Theresa, not just because of the pies, the laughing, or even those cute slippers you were selling, but your Spirit and your Belief in something much higher than man. Now that I think back, that's what got you through.

I love you "T",

Sandra Johnson

***

Theresa,

You are someone that I consider my sister. The guidance that you have given me has helped my life and continues to. You are my mentor. When you were diagnosed with cancer I prayed and prayed, but I knew in my heart the Lord was not ready to take you from us. He knew that your work here was not done. You are his personal soldier. To help you with this battle, I knew I had to help you fight. I didn't have to think about it. I grabbed my holistic book gave it to you to look up recipes. I brought in beets, carrots, ginger roots and apples. I started blending them together and bringing it to work. You really didn't like the Sperlina juice, but you drank it anyway. You know that you are loved by so many people. May you continue to be blessed and may you continue to bless others.

I love you sister girl,

Terrina Harris-Sanders

***

Theresa,

Life hands us obstacles that we must learn to overcome. There are few people who choose to look at these obstacles as a test; Theresa did. What Theresa Hart has endured these past few years has made her stronger, more determined, and as patient and loving as she was before her illness. She has shown me that the obstacle that was handed to her was nothing more than that, an obstacle, a hurdle if you may, that she was determined to climb over. Needless to say my friend Theresa passed the test and was an inspiration to all involved in her life during her illness and now during her recovery. Theresa is someone who I hold dear as a friend, teacher and hero.

Love,

Kelley McCoskey

***

Theresa,

Prior to Theresa's illness she helped guide me through a crisis of faith. Her faith is so strong and solid, that it helped her and her family deal with her illness. She also helped all her friends during this time of crisis, more as if we were ill and she was comforting us. Theresa is a very strong woman who helps her family, friends and neighbors. She started a Girls' Club with I think six "young ladies" and it grew and grew. That was so successful she and her husband started a Boys' Club with "young men"—all from the neighborhood. From working full time, being a Deaconess in her church, taking care of her ladies and young men; cooking for her immediate and extended family, among all the other things she did—I often asked her how she did it. She shrugged and said, "I just do it" and things get done. Let go and let God! That is not just a saying, it is the way she lives her life.

Dorothy Winhiemer

***

Theresa,

How do you encourage a friend who is and has been my biggest supporter since I decided to give my life to Christ? When I say, "I can't," she says "the devil is a liar" and then begins the short sermon about the gifts of God. I dubbed her Pastor/Mother Theresa Hart, long before her trial sermon. I remember when you and my adopted church family (Uncle Kevin, Cousin Nikki and "lil" cousin Jack) took their hiatus; even when you told me your family wasn't coming back to NLT, it never actually sunk in. I even told you on more than a few occasions, "You'll be back," I knew you would, you loved the church too much to just walk away. When you told me about your illness, I remember thinking that this sickness is not unto death, but to glorify God! So now you're here with your "first" book, expressing like only you can. To God be the glory for the things He has done. I wish you much success and many blessings. For eyes have not seen, ears have not heard...I am so proud of you.

Love you much,

Gretchen Mitchell

***

Theresa,

What you have been through I would not have wished on anyone, but God allowed it knowing that you could handle it and still praise Him through it. Whenever I saw you, I remember thinking, "What a warrior she is!" You never looked as though you were going through. This book was birthed because of who you are in Christ. There's no doubt souls will be touched and you will be successful.

Your friend and sister in Christ.

I love you,

Denise

***

Dear Theresa,

I am writing this letter as a friend and sister. I would first like to thank you for being the wonderful friend that you are. We have cried and laughed together over the years. I am so proud of you! You are an awesome woman; you have endured many life challenges and have always come through eloquently. Your determination and drive are what keeps me going in my moments of trial. As you embark on becoming the next "Bestselling Author" I salute you for all your accomplishments and wish you continued peace and blessings in everything you do! A trusted friend is so difficult to find, I am glad we found each other!

Pamela Miles

***

My Dearest Theresa,

When I found out that you had cancer, I became sad and worried. However, knowing that you are a child of God, and that He is always there watching over you, I knew and felt that you would overcome it! I saw you in your worst, and then I saw you getting better. I prayed every night and day for your well-being. I thank God for your greatest recovery and remission from this enemy called cancer. I'm very happy to see that you are continuously doing well each day and being strong in the Lord - who brought you through it all. I'm grateful to still have you here with us. May God keep on blessing you and your family always.

Sincerely,

DJenny DeMorcy

***

Theresa,

Living through cancer with a smile and a positive attitude – What an inspiration you are to all who were in contact with you at work. You did your job with such a positive attitude. None of us doubted the outcome of complete recovery.

Betty Ann McKenna

To my beloved sister,

"Survived my darkest hour, my faith kept me alive. I picked myself back up, hold my head up high, I was not built to break, I didn't know my own strength!" ~ Whitney Houston.

If this book had to be accompanied with a CD song to back it up, it would definitely be, "I Didn't Know My Own Strength". That song and the powerful testimony that lies within this book, says it ALL, sis! And do know that I am so glad that you don't look like what you've been through. Congratulations on the accomplishment of this long awaited endeavor, Evangelist Hart. I promise you, the only thing that the readers will hear throughout the entire book is, "I was not built to break!"

I Believe God,

Evangelist Hilgra Hatcher

***

Theresa,

As the deer panteth for the water so does my soul longeth after thee. You alone are my heart's desire and I long to worship thee. You alone are my strength and shield, you alone make my heart stand still. You alone are my heart's desire and I long to worship thee, And I long to worship thee.

This was the song I sang when I visited you when you where recovering from your first chemo treatment. You kept saying, "The pain, Jamesetta, the pain…" The more I sang the song to you, the more it seemed it brought you comfort while I sat at the edge of your bed. It is so funny how God operates, Theresa. I remember when you first heard that you had to have chemotherapy. You called me and said, "Jamesetta, I need a women gyn-oncologist." I said, "Okay, let's pray." At the time, you didn't tell me any names that you were given on a list. I sat at my desk and prayed and asked God to lead you. My co-worker who is also a breast cancer survivor and a faith based believer came in the hallway to go to the bathroom. I said to her, "My sister was diagnosed with breast cancer and I need a doctor." She looked at me with tears in her eyes and said, "Here is a doctor. She is amazing and will take care of your sister." When I called you and told you, you let me know that somebody had already given you her name. We knew from then that God was in control.

Theresa, I don't know if you know this, but at that time you were strength in the eyes of many. Your illness became real to people because until you have somebody close to you that goes through breast cancer, you cannot relate. When I sat there through one of your chemo sessions I looked at you as the epitome of God's strength. No matter what was said or done, you believed God.

Hey, remember before all of this, we went to have pizza when you first got diagnosed, before you even went to go see the doctors; when you couldn't believe what was going on and what you were hearing? Remember, the scripture Randy gave you - the scripture that Pastor Hunter preached that Sunday, "Simon Peter, Simon Peter the enemy has come to sift thee as wheat but I have prayed for you, that when you recover strengthen your brethren."

We were basking in the Word as we ate that pizza. By the way I haven't had pizza that good since that day. We ate saying,

"Hey, if God told Peter that God prayed for him, what has He done for us? Look what Peter was, look at what he did and God told him that he was going to go through, but that He prayed for him.

What better prayer could there be to have Jesus pray for you, we concluded. Girl, we were almost tore up in that restaurant that day with all the praise and worship we were having; we were having church. When we left there, girl, you were encouraged to go through whatever you needed to go through.

So know that with this book you are doing just what God had intended for you to do, to strengthen the brethren. God knows that there are others that are going to go through this sifting in their life. They are going to be able to pick up this book and be strengthened. Praise God for the victory, Theresa.

Love you,

Jamesetta, "Prophetess"

***

Theresa,

In our lifetime, we have to deal with the choices we make; the choices that are made for us and the everyday ups and downs that are just life. The phrase that is important to me and I apply it to everything is, "Life is 10% what happens to you and 90% how you react to it." I don't remember who said it, but it's my first line of thought. People have often said to me, "How do you stay so calm?" I prefer to spend my 90% reaction time taking a step back and working out a solution instead of emotionally decompensating and stressing out. Best wishes to you and remember you are too blessed to be stressed.

Aretha

***

The Clark Family Sentiment

Ecclesiastes 3:1 states, "To every *thing there is* a season, and a time to every purpose under the heaven." Oh, how great is our God, which in His infinite wisdom has purposed and planned the Hart Family & the Clark Family to connect in the sweetest fellowship ever, the body of Christ.

It has been a joy, an exuberant legacy of our families who have known the importance of family and friends, and most assuredly God, being in the midst. We share family experiences, as we reflect on our good days and some bad days. However, when we were in the fiery furnace you stood and prayed with us and when you were in the lion's den we stood and prayed with you. We exalt the name of our Lord, and declare we will bless the Lord, at all times, and His Praises shall continually be in our mouths. (Psalm 34:1)

As we continue on our journey in Christ, one will face struggle, pain and certainly indecision. The Holy Spirit has guided you to demonstrate love, patience, and care, always utilizing the power of prayer. We love you so much, and we know that this sentiment will edify and encourage. Words could never truly express the joy, the love and the gratitude we feel for you. We want to encourage you and pray that everything that God has laid to your charge, will flourish, multiply, and enlarge your territory. Be encouraged. The sacrifices that you have made will never be forgotten. We can simply say with conviction that we know you as the Hart Foundation because you are rooted and grounded in Jesus. May God keep you and continue to use you as shining lights for His Glory. "The LORD bless thee, and keep thee: The LORD make his face shine upon thee, and be gracious unto thee: The LORD lift up his countenance upon thee, and give thee peace."(Numbers 6: 24-26)

Forever Love,

Darold and Veronica Clark

***

Theresa,

We have known you for several years and we have found you to be a very caring and giving person and we are lucky to be able to call you a good friend. I was a volunteer at your mentoring program and in spite of your cancer battle, you still found time to continue with the program and always seem to put your kids ahead of yourself. Theresa Hart, you are a very strong person and are truly an inspiration to us all. The lesson we can learn from you is that, you can survive anything as long as you have your faith, family and good friends around you. We wish you good health in the many years to come.

Kim and Michael Lewis

***

Dear Theresa,

It is because of our Lord and Savior Jesus Christ that I am a witness of your blessed life. I am a witness of your trials and your tribulations in which you have weathered them all. You were in the fiery furnace of affliction, but God. And not because of any great thing you've done, but it is because of Him - the one who suffered, bled and died for us all - Jesus. Girl, you are soaring with the eagles and I am rejoicing. The scripture says to rejoice with them that rejoice! May you continue to soar with the eagles - what a great Christian leader, wife, mother and friend you are. Psalms 27 says, "Wait on the Lord: be of good courage, and he shall strengthen thine heart: wait, I say, on the Lord." Isaiah 40:28-31 states, "Hast thou not known? hast thou not heard, that the everlasting God, the Lord, the Creator of the ends of the earth, fainteth not, neither is weary? there is no searching of his understanding. He giveth power to the faint, and to them that have no might he increaseth strength. Even the youths shall faint and be weary, and the young men shall utterly fall. But they that wait upon the Lord shall renew their strength; they shall mount up with wings as eagles, they shall run, and not be weary; and they shall walk, and not faint." To God be all the glory for the great things He has done and continues to do in your life.

You've waited and He has done it. He has restored you, my friend. Congratulations on your ministry of writing. I know that this work shall bless many. For it is out of our suffering that a great work is birthed. I believe God!

Love,

Elder Yolanda R. Collins

Theresa,

I have known you for over 20 years as your Primary Care Physician. You were diagnosed with Breast Cancer by me in 2008. Your courage, endurance, perseverance, and fighting spirit are exemplary to each and every one of us.

Dr. Suresh Patel

***

Dearest Theresa,

"One Survivor to Another"

I haven't read your book yet, but your life has been an open book. I've watched you weather the storms and you have been a sustaining force during your battle with the dreadful disease of cancer and the debilitating effects of the chemotherapy. You've walked me through a dark tunnel of despair until I came out on the other side; your prayers and encouragement helped me to make it through. It is because of your life that I eagerly await the release of your awesome book. To God be the Glory!

Evangelist Tina Gates,

Author of An Unexpected Journey and spiritual mother

***

Evangelist Theresa Hart,

I have known you for over 19 years. You are a wonderful person to be around and with. When I got the news that you had cancer "OMG" [OH MY GOD]! It took me down. One day I was on the bus and said "Lord, I don't ask you for much, I need you to work this out for Theresa". These scriptures came to me Exodus 15:26 and 1 Peter 2:24. I know prayer works. "Lord, whatever you do please do it for Evangelist Hart. Her family needs her." I wasn't able to get to the hospital or your home, but I know prayer can go where I can't. Theresa, you went through breast cancer, chemotherapy, and radiation and this sickness still did not break you! Look at what the Lord has done for you!

Love you,

Minister Isaac Conyers

***

Theresa,

I take this opportunity to thank God for you, my sister, Minister Theresa Hart. Look what the Lord has done. Mastermind. He makes no mistakes for He knows the way we take. All things happen for a reason and a season. So glad to be a part of your journey through life; time and space will not permit me to elaborate the way I feel in my heart, but know that eyes have not seen neither have ears heard, nor has it entered into the hearts of man the things God has in store for US as WE walk this road TOGETHER. I'm so proud of you.

Much Love,

First Lady Doreen Figueroa

Evangelist Theresa Hart,

You are one of the most indomitable and enduring individuals that I have had the pleasure of knowing. Your love of God and spirit of integrity has left an indelible mark in my quest for excellence in spiritual pursuits. Your zeal and passion for God is what has anchored you through the many tumultuous storms in your life, particularly your latest struggle. You have a victorious soul and a "Can Do" attitude that epitomizes the strength and purposes our Heavenly Father has placed in us all. Nothing is insurmountable for you, Theresa, for you have completely and totally put your trust in God and has laid your life in His hands. As a prayer partner your prayers have often rendered Satan speechless as you cried on behalf of others and touched the heart of God. One thing is for sure, you will stand in the gap. Your tender heart for souls is what fuels you the most. Your ministry is global in concept and intimate in affiliation. You bring to life the scripture "And of some have compassion, making a difference:" Jude 1:22. Life is just better when you are around and I'm sure these few pages will validate everything I just mentioned. To my sister in Christ, I thank you.

Lovingly Submitted,

Evangelist Tammy Vaughn

***

Theresa Hart and I first met in 1996 when she worked as a clerical temp for our hospital program. Theresa's intelligence and organization skills were apparent from the very first day of her employment. As we worked together I could also see Theresa's drive and motivation. This was a formula for success. Theresa was encouraged to take advantage of her educational opportunities with our hospital's Union. She followed through and is now a college graduate. In addition, Theresa recently became a minister and continues to follow through with her religious calling. Theresa has fostered her church's food bank program and mentored the young women of her church. None of this came without cost. Theresa was exhausted but prayed for strength to do it all. Her prayers were answered. Theresa is a loving, supportive wife and mother, proud of her successful young daughter and teenage son. Theresa is also a breast cancer survivor. Theresa Hart is a fighter and a winner and a true inspiration.

Maryann Riccardo

***

About the Author

Theresa Hart

Theresa Hart is passionate about helping people overcome obstacles to live productive and extraordinary lives.

Formerly addicted to substance abuse, Theresa knows the ins and outs of struggling to make her life better. By applying perseverance and faith she has steadily overcome life's trials.

Early in her career, Theresa worked in a substance abuse and MICA/AIDS program. This position prompted her to obtain a degree. Theresa now holds a B.A. in Social Services and works in the Department of Psychiatry. She is also a minister at her local church.

Theresa and her husband Kevin have been married over 30 years and make their home in Elmont, NY with their two children; Nicole and Kevin, Jr.

You may contact Theresa at authortheresahart@gmail.com. You may also visit her website at www.authortheresahart.com.

www.ingramcontent.com/pod-product-compliance
Lightning Source LLC
Chambersburg PA
CBHW070756290326
41931CB00011BA/2041
9780615667775